How to Pass

SECOND EDITION

NATIONAL 5

Music

Joe McGowan

**HODDER
GIBSON**

AN HACHETTE UK COMPANY

The Publishers would like to thank the following for permission to reproduce copyright material:

CD tracks (see list, pp. 86–88): 'Tomorrow' (from *Annie*): Warner Chappell (performance by Sotogrande International School); Mozart's Piano Concerto no. 21 in C Major, K467, 'Elvira Madigan' (movement 2, *Andante*): Naxos; Beethoven's Symphony no. 9 (movement 2, *Molto vivace*): Warner Chapell; Bach's *Air on a G string*: The Pickwick Group Ltd; Verdi's 'La Donna e Mobile' (from *Rigoletto*): Countdown Media; *Go Tell it on the Mountain*: Blue Mountain Music; Purcell's *Music for a While*: The Pickwick Group Ltd; Wagner's 'Sailors' Chorus' (from *The Flying Dutchman*): ONE MEDIA iP Ltd; Handel's *Menuet* (from 'Water Music': suite in F major): The Pickwick Group Ltd; *Cancion para un niño*: Mr Bongo Worldwide Ltd; Strauss's *Emperor's Waltz*, op. 437: Countdown Media; Wagner's Pilgrim's Chorus 'Beglückt darf nun': ONE MEDIA iP Ltd.

All licensing rights by permission MCPS/PRS

Photo credits p. 7 © kameramann/Fotolia; **p. 11** © Mr Twister/Fotolia; **p. 29** © Andy Dean/Fotolia; **p. 45** © auremar/Fotolia; **p. 58** © jacek_kadaj/Fotolia.

Acknowledgements Composing advice (p. 29) and composing review information (p. 57) taken from the SQA N5 Course Specification 2017–18 session (July 2017) PDF used by permission copyright © Scottish Qualifications Authority

Special thanks to Jenny Reynolds, Derek Norval, Chloe Lawrence, and Emma Isola and Kerry Wickersham (Sotogrande International School).

Every effort has been made to trace all copyright holders, but if any have been inadvertently overlooked the Publishers will be pleased to make the necessary arrangements at the first opportunity.

Although every effort has been made to ensure that website addresses are correct at time of going to press, Hodder Gibson cannot be held responsible for the content of any website mentioned in this book. It is sometimes possible to find a relocated web page by typing in the address of the home page for a website in the URL window of your browser.

Hachette UK's policy is to use papers that are natural, renewable and recyclable products and made from wood grown in well-managed forests and other controlled sources. The logging and manufacturing processes are expected to conform to the environmental regulations of the country of origin.

Orders: please contact Bookpoint Ltd, 130 Park Drive, Milton Park, Abingdon, Oxon OX14 4SE. Telephone: (44) 01235 827720. Fax: (44) 01235 400454. Lines are open 9.00–5.00, Monday to Friday, with a 24-hour message answering service. Visit our website at www.hoddereducation.co.uk. If you have queries or questions that aren't about an order, you can contact us at hoddergibson@hodder.co.uk

© Joe McGowan 2018

First published in 2018 by
Hodder Gibson, an imprint of Hodder Education,
An Hachette UK Company
211 St Vincent Street
Glasgow G2 5QY

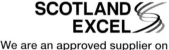

SCOTLAND EXCEL

We are an approved supplier on the Scotland Excel framework.

Schools can find us on their procurement system as:
Hodder & Stoughton Limited t/a Hodder Gibson.

Impression number	5 4 3 2
Year	2022 2021 2020 2019

Cover photo © vasvas/123RF
Illustrations by Aptara, Inc.
Typeset in Cronos Pro 13/15 by Aptara, Inc.
Printed in India
A catalogue record for this title is available from the British Library
ISBN: 978 1 5104 2104 2

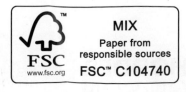

MIX
Paper from responsible sources
FSC™ C104740
FSC
www.fsc.org

Contents

Introduction

Welcome!

Wouldn't it be great to have a really smart study partner on hand whenever you needed help with any aspect of your National 5 Music course – a person who could also guide you through revision when the final exams and assessments are approaching?

Yes? Well, the following pages are packed with information, exercises and top advice to make everything easier and, hopefully, more enjoyable. There are also two companion websites with supplementary material for that extra help that will keep you especially well informed: **www.hoddergibson. co.uk/updatesandextras** and **www.jm-education.com**.

The author who put all this together is an experienced teacher and professional musician who wants you to pass as much as you do. So, now that you have your really smart study partner sorted out, let's get started!

The National 5 Music qualification

National 5 Music is intended to be an enjoyable course that provides you with knowledge, which will increase your understanding and appreciation of music all through life. This knowledge can be divided into four main components.

1   Musical literacy

Musical literacy, or music theory, involves the symbols, note values, rhythms and so on that make up music notation – the written 'language' of music. Just as in story writing, where the better you understand spoken language the more interesting your story is likely to be, so your achievements in music will improve if you learn to speak *its* unique language.

Chapter 2 contains a reference for all the music notation you need to understand at National 5 level.

2   Listening

Music is communicated through sound. Understanding what you hear (listening) is fundamental to all areas of musical activity, including composing and performing. National 5 Music requires you to listen to many different types of music and identify what you hear by indicating the musical concepts present – these are the elements that make up different types of music. The first chapter in this book covers all the concepts you need to understand by the end of the course, when you will be assessed in the form of a Listening test paper that lasts 45 minutes. A specimen test question paper is provided for you in Chapter 3, and another can be accessed on YouTube from the jm-education website, **www.jm-education.com**.

3　Composing

National 5 Music will introduce you to creating original music (composing). Throughout the course you will learn various composing techniques and processes, then demonstrate your knowledge of these by creating your own composition in any style/genre, lasting between 1 minute and 2 minutes 30 seconds.

For this composing assignment, you will work in close consultation with your class teacher who will guide you along the way, helping you get it ready for the final assessment, which is carried out by an external examiner.

Chapter 4 takes you step by step through a number of useful techniques which demonstrate methods for composing both instrumental and vocal music.

4　Performing

Playing or singing music (performing) is an important part of National 5 Music, and carries **50%** of the total available marks. You can perform on **either** two musical instruments of your choice, **or** a musical instrument and voice. You can perform **solo**, in a **group** or a combination of both. Help on this part of the course is given in Chapter 5.

At the end of your course you will perform a prepared programme of music lasting between 8 and 8½ minutes, which will be assessed by a visiting examiner. You must play each of your two selected instruments (or instrument and voice) for a minimum of **2 minutes** within the total programme. In all areas of performing, playing expressively is as important as technical skill alone. Your teacher will help you choose appropriate music for this programme, and further guidance can be found on the National 5 Music pages of the Scottish Qualifications Authority website **www.sqa.org.uk/sqa/47391.html**.

Solo performing

Here you should play or sing a selection of **contrasting** pieces of music, which may include some **improvisation**. You will be assessed on the standard of music chosen and how well you play it.

Group performing

This can involve playing in a band or as part of an ensemble. For example, you might be the lead vocalist in a rock, folk or jazz band, the violinist in a string quartet, or the trumpet player in a wind ensemble. Your programme can include both solo and group performances on one instrument, providing you perform for at least 2 minutes on the other instrument (or voice).

Assessment for your final grade

There are three main assessment components:

1 **Musical performance.** This carries **50%** of the total available marks and is split evenly between your two performances (see table on the right).

2 **Listening test question paper.** This carries **35%** of the total available marks. The question paper, which is based on musical excerpts, tests your knowledge of the various musical styles and concepts you will have studied throughout your course.

3 **Composing assignment.** This carries **15%** of the total available marks. **10%** of these marks are awarded for the composition itself, and the remaining **5%** is for your written account of the various decisions you've made, the processes involved etc. in its creation. You are also asked to identify any strengths and/or areas that might need some improvement.

See the table for how this translates to actual marks.

Component	Marks	Scaled mark
Component 1: question paper	40	35
Component 2: assignment Marks are divided as follows —	30	15
composing music	20	
composing review	10	
Component 3: performance — instrument 1	30	25
Component 4: performance — instrument 2	30	25

How to use this book

How to Pass National 5 Music can function both as a textbook to help you during the course and as a revision guide towards its conclusion. Working through the chapters and exercises carefully will ensure that you gather all the knowledge and reference material you need to succeed.

We'll begin in Chapter 1 by reviewing the musical concepts you need to know at this level, since an understanding of these concepts is essential for all areas of the course, including **Listening**, **Musical literacy** and **Composing**.

Throughout the book you will find a range of exercises, information and tips designed to help you learn quickly and painlessly. The book also includes a complete specimen listening test, similar to the exam you will sit at the end of the course. You will even have the opportunity to devise some of your own listening exercises.

Key-2-success words

Important words – your 'key-2-success' words – are shown throughout the book in two colours, **red** and **blue**. These are the key words that can be used in an internet search to find out more about a concept or a related topic. Those in **red** are the important musical concepts that you must understand for National 5 Music, and those in **blue** are words related to a concept or an aspect of music that will improve your knowledge. The blue words also indicate pieces of music in which particular musical concepts can be found.

For example, in the **Suggested listening** lists in Chapter 1, information appears like this:

Concept	Piece title	Composer (Performer)
Classical	Symphony no. 5 in C minor, op. 67	Beethoven (Royal Philharmonic Orchestra)

The main concepts are shown in **red** followed by, in **blue**, the title of a piece of music that is an example of the concept. Next comes the composer and/or performer's name (in brackets). Searching for this information on a website that provides music recordings will locate Beethoven's 5th Symphony, while doing the same on an encyclopaedia type site (or in a general Google or Yahoo search), will find detailed information on this symphony. Simply typing '**Classical** music,' '**Symphony**' or '**Beethoven**' will of course also produce a lot of information about Classical music, the symphony, and the life and music of this particular composer, should you want to do further research.

The exercises

This book uses three main kinds of exercises to help you revise and understand as you work through each chapter. They can be carried out by individuals or groups of students.

Suggested listening

Concept	Piece title	Composer (Performer(s))
Classical	Symphony no. 5 in C minor, op. 67	Beethoven
	The Marriage of Figaro (opera)	Mozart
Waulking song	Skye Waulking Song	Traditional (Capercaillie)
	Gaelic Waulking Song	Traditional (Sgioba Luaidh)

'Suggested listening' lists pieces of music that are examples of, or feature, the musical concepts you need to know at National 5 level. Your colour-coded key-2-success words (see page vi) play a vital role in these lists. For space reasons, this book only includes suggested listening lists for National 5 **STYLES** concepts. However, a complete set of lists (including those for National 3 and National 4) can be found in the supplementary material for Chapter 1 at www. hoddergibson.co.uk/updatesandextras or www.jm-education.com.

CD exercises and musical examples

The CD accompanying this book contains musical excerpts for use with the **specimen listening test** question paper in Chapter 3, and examples for the **composing** exercises in Chapter 4. There are also two extra tracks: one featuring a piece of instrumental music composed on a music **sequencer**, and the other a song written and performed by a teenage music student. You can see how both of these were put together, step by step, in the supplementary composing workshops at **www.jm-education.com**.

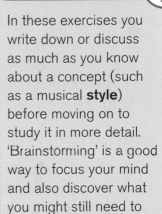

Brainstorm !

In these exercises you write down or discuss as much as you know about a concept (such as a musical **style**) before moving on to study it in more detail. 'Brainstorming' is a good way to focus your mind and also discover what you might still need to learn.

Things to consider when discussing each musical concept include the main characteristic(s) of each concept and, where appropriate, the names of any particular songs or pieces you know that contain or represent a concept, together with their composer(s). Your descriptions don't need to be very detailed – single words or brief explanations might be enough. For definitions of each concept, or just to refresh your memory, refer to the glossary section at the end of the book.

Activity time ✏

These exercises, based on the musical concepts, involve practical listening and composing activities. They include explanation of how to create tests for your fellow music students, and how to get 'hands on' with the book's guidance.

Extra help

Glossary of musical concepts

The glossary at the back of the book gives definitions of each musical concept. There is a tick-box beside each one – these are for you to tick when you understand the meaning of each concept, or for your teacher to indicate those concepts he or she wants you to learn.

Online help

A comprehensive selection of suggested listening examples for use in Chapter 1 can be found on the Hodder Gibson website (**www.hoddergibson.co.uk/updatesandextras**). Personal advice and online tuition is available at **www.yourmusicmentor.com**.

This book's main companion website (**www.jm-education.com**) includes a lot of free supplementary resource material for teachers and students, including suggested listening lists for National 3, National 4 and National 5 concepts, additional composing material with two full songwriting and composing workshops (see CD tracks 34 and 35), and other pieces of helpful information. The website will be reviewed and updated whenever required to reflect any curriculum changes.

Tip maestro

The book's resident music adviser, tip maestro, pops up frequently to offer little bits of advice and helpful information.

Concepts at work

These give a little more information on those concepts that might need extra explanation (such as **cadences** and **chord progressions**), illustrating their function – or how they 'work' – in pieces of music.

How to approach music

Music often has complex-sounding words for concepts that are actually quite easy to understand. For example, **anacrusis** only means that a piece of music doesn't begin on the first beat of the bar; **counterpoint** describes music that has two or more different melodies sounding together in **harmony**; and imitative **polyphony** just indicates that a group of singers are imitating each other's vocal lines. Remember: just because a concept sounds complex doesn't mean that it is.

We learn more effectively by taking in small amounts at a time, absorbing manageable pieces of information as we work towards digesting an entire course of study. People who 'eat' knowledge in this way remember and understand what they have learned and grow confident in their ability, whereas those who try to cram it all in close to the exam get stressed out and quickly forget information. This book has a 'one bite at a time' approach. Whether you are learning concepts or composing music, you will succeed if you don't become daunted by the size of the task and take it all in small pieces.

When working on any course, having your work well organised – categorised neatly in a folder – makes for easy, stress-free study. You will avoid frustration when you want to find something and your revision will be faster. Good organisation will even help you develop confidence in your own academic ability.

Musical concepts

In this chapter you will revise all the musical concepts you need to know. Musical concepts are the various elements (melody, instruments, rhythm, harmony etc.) that make up a piece of music. The chapter works through a series of units that focus on five broad categories of concepts, outlined below. Using the *Suggested listening* lists and *Activity time* exercises you will explore each concept and steadily increase your understanding of them all.

The five broad categories of musical concepts are:

1 **Style** (the general type of music – for example, **classical**, **rock**, **jazz**, **blues**)
2 **Melody** (the tune or tunes in a piece of music) and **harmony** (the notes and/or **chords** that accompany a melody)
3 **Rhythm** (the different time durations of musical notes and rests in a piece of music) and **tempo** (the speed of the music)
4 **Texture**, **structure** and **form** (the way a musical composition is constructed; the types of musical concepts it uses)
5 **Timbre** (the sounds that musical instruments – including voice – produce either individually or when playing together in different combinations) and **dynamics** (the volume levels in a piece of music).

We will start with the musical concepts for National 5, followed by those from National 4 and National 3 that you also need to know. To see the complete series of suggested listening lists for the course and supplementary material for each chapter go to **www.hoddergibson. co.uk/updatesandextras** or **www.jm-education.com**.

National 5 musical concepts

Unit 1 National 5 STYLE concepts

Symphony	Waulking song
Gospel	Gaelic psalm
Classical	Aria
Pibroch	Chorus
Celtic rock	Minimalist
Bothy ballad	Indian

Brainstorm 1 !

Write down or discuss with your classmates what you know about these **STYLE** concepts and think about whether you would be able to recognise each one by ear.

Listening observation chart

STYLE	Composer/performer	Compositions/performances	Concepts/instruments/other characteristics
Symphony	Mozart Beethoven Mahler	Symphonies 1–41 Symphonies 1–9 Symphonies 1–10	Large instrumental work for orchestra in several movements (normally three to five). Each movement has a different character and tempo.
Gospel	Marvin Sapp Traditional John Newton	The Best in Me Oh Happy Day Amazing Grace	Religious vocal music influenced by negro spirituals and hymns. Sung by soloists or, more commonly, large choirs. Livelier than other religious music such as hymns.
Classical	Haydn Mozart Beethoven	The Creation The Magic Flute Moonlight Sonata	1750–1820 (approximately). Symmetry is important in the structure of classical compositions, with more expression and larger orchestra than in Baroque music that came before it. Piano and clarinet are developed.

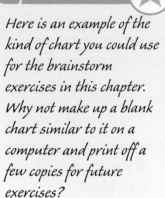

Tip maestro ★

Here is an example of the kind of chart you could use for the brainstorm exercises in this chapter. Why not make up a blank chart similar to it on a computer and print off a few copies for future exercises?

When you have completed the brainstorm exercise, refer below to the suggested listening examples for Unit 1. You may find it helpful to use an online source to find the suggested pieces of music.

Note: All other suggested listening lists can be located at **www.hoddergibson.co.uk/updatesandextras** or **www.jm-education.com**.

Suggested listening for Unit 1

Concept	Piece title	Composer (performer(s))
Symphony	No. 1 'Titan' No. 9 'The Choral' No. 9 'From the new world'	Mahler Beethoven Dvořák
Gospel	Put Your Hands Up – Praise Chant Nobody Greater, Searched all Over I Look to You	(Shane Forrester) (Va Shawn Mitchell) (Whitney Houston)
Classical	Symphony 94 Overture from 'The Marriage of Figaro' (opera) Für Elise	Haydn Mozart Beethoven
Pibroch	Lament pibroch piobaireachd ceol mor. Drone (chanter) bagpipes Pibroch – Clan Ranald's March to Edinburgh (Clàrsach) Sheila's Jig	(Duncan MacRae) Traditional Traditional

 ⇨

Concept	Piece title	Composer (performer(s))
Celtic rock	Scotland	(Wolfstone)
	Caledonia	(Highlander Celtic Rock Band)
	Loch Lomond	(Prydein) or (Runrig)
Bothy ballad	The Keach in the Creel	Traditional (Ewan MacColl)
	MacPherson's Rant	Traditional (Davie Stewart)
	The Barnyards of Delgaty	Traditional (sung by Gaberlunzie)
Waulking song	Skye Waulking Song	Traditional (Capercaillie)
	Gaelic Waulking Song	Traditional (Sgioba Luaidh)
	Skye Waulking Song – 'My Father Sent me to the House of Sorrow'	Traditional (Karen Matheson)
Gaelic psalm	Moravia	Traditional
	Martyrs	Traditional (Isobel Ann Martin)
	Stroudwater (Psalm 46)	Traditional
Aria	Soave sia il Vento (from the opera 'Cosi Fan Tutte')	Mozart
	Nessun Dorma (from the opera 'Turandot')	Puccini
	Amor ti Vieta (from the opera 'Fedora')	Umberto Giordano
Chorus	Bridal Chorus 'Treulich geführt' (from the opera 'Lohengrin')	Wagner
	Gypsy Chorus (from the opera 'Il Trovatore')	Verdi
	Hallelujah Chorus (from the oratorio 'Messiah')	Handel
Minimalist	Shaker Loops	John Adams
	In C	Terry Riley
	The Hours	Philip Glass
Indian	Ancient Love	Anoushka Shankar
	Raag Hansaddhwani (Indian flute)	Pandit Hari
	Raag Yaman	Ustad Sultan Khan

Activity time 1

Set a listening test

Choose a few new pieces or excerpts of music based on National 5 **STYLE** concepts (perhaps sourced online) and play them to your fellow students to see if they can identify the concept that describes the **STYLE** of each one. They can do the same to test you, but of course by choosing the music for this exercise you will have already completed a listening exercise.

Note: You can carry out this type of listening exercise for each unit in this chapter.

Unit 2 National 5 MELODY/HARMONY concepts

Atonal	Tone/semitone
Cluster	Modulation
Chord progression (I, IV, V, VI major keys)	Contrary motion
Perfect cadence	Trill
Imperfect cadence	Syllabic
Inverted pedal	Melismatic
Chromatic	Countermelody
Whole-tone scale	Descant (voice)
Grace note	Pitch bend
Glissando	

Brainstorm 2

Write down or discuss with your classmates what you know about these **MELODY/HARMONY** concepts and think about whether you would be able to recognise each one by ear.

Concepts at work

Tone/semitone

For more information or study advice on **tones** and **semitones** see **National 5 musical literacy** on page 19 and the supplementary material for this unit at **www.jm-education.com**.

Chord progression

Chords I, IV, V and VI have been the principal chords used in all styles of Western music since about 1600. They commonly occur in popular songs from **rock 'n' roll**, **blues**, **rock**, **folk** and **pop** music as the catchy tunes of these styles are often built upon simple harmonic structures.

For more information or study advice on these chords see the Activity time exercises below and the supplementary material for this unit at **www.jm-education.com**.

Activity time 2

Identifying chords I, IV, V and VI in major keys by ear

To be able to identify the above chords by ear you must get used to hearing them. Try playing them over and over on a harmonic instrument such as a **keyboard**, **piano** or **guitar** until you begin to recognise the sound characteristic of each one. This sort of repetitive listening will help you to identify the chords when you hear them in a piece of music. After doing this you and your study partners can test each other's identification skills by having one person play the chords in various combinations while the others listen and try to identify the progression.

For help with choosing chord sequences see the supplementary material for this unit at **www.jm-education.com**.

Activity time 3

Identifying chords I, IV, V and VI in major keys by sight

Look at the printed music for a selection of popular songs and see if you can identify these chords at work. First, of course, you must know the key of each song in order to establish **chord I**, the 'key' chord. This will then allow you to identify **chords IV**, **V** and **VI**. Some songs may have other unfamiliar chords, others might use only **I**, **IV** and **V** (this is fairly common in simple **blues** and **rock 'n' roll** music). It is also possible that you will see 'altered' **I**, **IV** and **V** chords. For example, if **chord I** is **C major** you might see this altered to C9 or C maj7. Don't be confused by this. This is still basically a **C major chord**, just with an extra note added.

Activity time 4

Listen carefully for those concepts

Select a few pieces of music in different **styles** and listen out for the **MELODY/HARMONY** concepts listed on page 4. To make it easier, just select a few concepts to listen out for at first, and then gradually build up to the full list. You will find it helpful to make a listening chart similar to that used for the brainstorm exercises.

Note: You can carry out this type of listening exercise for other units in this chapter.

Suggested listening for Unit 2

When you have completed the brainstorm exercise, refer to the suggested listening examples for Unit 2 at www.hoddergibson.co.uk/updatesandextras or www.jm-education.com for examples of each of the above **MELODY/HARMONY** concepts.

Unit 3 National 5 TEXTURE/STRUCTURE/FORM concepts

Strophic	Ground bass
Binary – A B	Homophonic
Rondo (A B A C A ...) – episode	Polyphonic
Alberti bass	Contrapuntal
Walking bass	Coda

Brainstorm 3

Write down or discuss with your classmates what you know about these **TEXTURE/STRUCTURE/FORM** concepts and think about whether you would be able to recognise each one by ear.

Suggested listening for Unit 3

When you have completed the brainstorm exercise, refer to the suggested listening examples for Unit 3 at www.hoddergibson.co.uk/updatesandextras or www.jm-education.com for examples of each of the above TEXTURE/STRUCTURE/FORM concepts.

Activity time 5

Can you create a walking bass, Alberti bass and ground bass?

After listening to or looking at how these three bass accompaniments are structured, try composing a short example of each and test your study partner(s) by playing each one for them to identify.

If you don't yet have the playing skills, you could also write a short example of each type of bass accompaniment in music notation and see if other students can identify them by sight. For help with this exercise see the glossary in this book and the reference pages at **www.jm-education.com**.

Unit 4 National 5 TIMBRE/DYNAMICS concepts

Piccolo	Sitar
Oboe	Tabla
Bassoon	Arco
French horn	Pizzicato
Tuba	Con sordino
Viola	Flutter tonguing
Castanets	Rolls
Hi-hat cymbals	Reverb
Bongo drums	Mezzo-soprano
Clàrsach	Baritone
Bodhrán	A cappella

Brainstorm 4

Write down or discuss with your classmates what you know about these **TIMBRE/ DYNAMICS** concepts and think about whether you would be able to recognise each one by ear.

Suggested listening for Unit 4

When you have completed the brainstorm exercise, refer to the suggested listening examples for Unit 4 at www.hoddergibson. co.uk/updatesandextras or www.jm-education.com for examples of each of the above **TIMBRE/DYNAMICS** concepts.

Activity time 6

Identifying these concepts

Choose one piece of music from each of the **STYLES** below and see how many of the **TIMBRE/DYNAMICS** concepts studied in this unit you can identify. To help remind you, the concepts to listen out for appear in **red**.

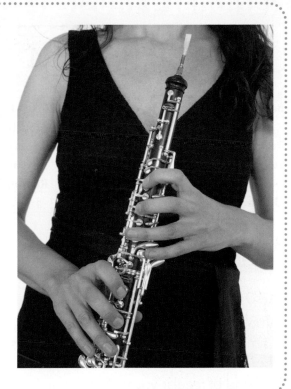

- **Orchestral music** (such as **symphonies, concertos**) **piccolo**; **oboe**; **bassoon**; **French horn**; **tuba**; **viola**; **arco**; **pizzicato**; **con sordino**; **flutter tonguing**; **rolls**
- **Flamenco music castanets**; **a cappella**
- **Scottish traditional/folk music clàrsach**
- **Irish traditional (Celtic) music bodhrán**
- **Latin-American Music bongo drums**
- **Rock, jazz and popular music hi-hat cymbals**; **reverb**
- **Indian music sitar**; **tabla**
- **Vocal music** (such as **arias** from an **opera**) **mezzo-soprano**; **baritone**; **a cappella**

Unit 5 National 5 RHYTHM/ TEMPO Concepts

Rubato	Cross rhythms
Ritardando	Compound time – 6/8, 9/8, 12/8
Moderato	

Brainstorm 5

Write down or discuss with your classmates what you know about these **RHYTHM/TEMPO** concepts and think about whether you would be able to recognise each one by ear.

Activity time 7

Improvise your way to understanding

A good way to strengthen your understanding of concepts or techniques is to get some hands-on experience *playing* them. For example, using the notes of a familiar musical scale you could improvise phrases in a moderate **tempo** (**moderato**) that are in **compound time** and have sections containing **rubato** and **ritardando** (both of which are quite common in improvised music).

To get experience with **cross rhythms** why not ask one of your fellow students to play a simple passage of music while you improvise a **cross rhythm** (in the same key) over it?

Note: You can carry out this type of improvising exercise for other units in this chapter.

Suggested listening for Unit 5

When you have completed the brainstorm exercise, refer to the suggested listening examples for Unit 5 at www. hoddergibson.co.uk/ updatesandextras or www.jm-education.com for examples of each of the above RHYTHM/ TEMPO concepts.

National 4 musical concepts

Unit 6 National 4 STYLE concepts

Baroque	Scots ballad
Ragtime	Mouth music
Romantic	Reggae
Swing	African music
Concerto	Rapping
Opera	

Brainstorm 6

Write down or discuss with your classmates what you know about these **STYLE** concepts and think about whether you would be able to recognise each one by ear.

Activity time 8

Rap it all up!

After listening carefully to a few examples of **rap** music, try composing a simple rap song of your own. Choose a subject you feel strongly about then write a few lines of text about it. Don't worry about writing the kind of regular vocal phrases you find in other songs. In rap music you have much more freedom to make the words 'fit' the beat. When you have your text, try saying the words out loud to a steady beat and listen as your rap song emerges. You might go on to add more instrumental accompaniment or sound loops to the beat and really build your work into something special.

Suggested listening for Unit 6

When you have completed the brainstorm exercise, refer to the suggested listening examples for Unit 6 at www.hoddergibson.co.uk/updatesandextras or www.jm-education.com for examples of each of the above STYLE concepts.

Unit 7 National 4 MELODY/HARMONY concepts

Major/minor (tonality)	Scale
Drone	Pentatonic scale
Broken chord/Arpeggio	Octave
Chord progression — chords I, IV and V (major keys)	Vamp
	Scat singing
Change of key	Ornament
Pedal	

Suggested listening for Unit 7

When you have completed the brainstorm exercise, refer to the suggested listening examples for Unit 7 at www.hoddergibson.co.uk/updatesandextras or www.jm-education.com for examples of each of the above MELODY/HARMONY concepts.

Brainstorm 7

Write down or discuss with your classmates what you know about these **MELODY/HARMONY** concepts and think about whether you would be able to recognise each one by ear.

Concepts at work

Super fast concept reference …

★ **Scat** singing is mainly associated with **jazz** music.

★ A **vamp** can be found in **rock 'n' roll** and **jazz**.

★ The **pentatonic scale** is used in **rock**, **jazz**, **blues**, **rock 'n' roll** and some **folk music**.

★ **Chords I, IV and V** are fundamental to **blues** and **rock 'n' roll**.

★ **Ornaments** are a feature of **Baroque** music.

★ A **drone** is often used in Scottish and Celtic music.

★ **Major/minor tonality**, **broken chords/arpeggios** and **changes of key** can occur in any style of music.

Activity time 9

Sharpen those listening skills

Choose a selection of the above concepts and, one at a time, play or sing them for your fellow students to identify. This exercise is useful whether you are performing or listening as it will help you focus on the unique character of each concept and become more familiar with its sound.

Note: You can take turns at this type of exercise, and of course try it with different concepts in other units in this chapter.

Unit 8 National 4 RHYTHM/TEMPO concepts

Syncopation	Anacrusis
Scotch snap	Andante
Strathspey	Accelerando
Jig	Rallentando
Simple time – 2/4, 3/4, 4/4	A tempo
Compound time	Dotted rhythms

Brainstorm 8

Write down or discuss with your classmates what you know about these **RHYTHM/TEMPO** concepts and think about whether you would be able to recognise each one by ear.

Activity time 10

Sharpen those observation skills

All of the concepts in this unit can be seen in musical scores. Using an online resource that lets you view such scores, study as much music as you can until you have identified at least one example of each concept.

Note: You can also use this as a test for your fellow students and of course the exercise can be carried out in other units in this chapter.

Activity time 11

Concepts in Scottish music

Choose a number of pieces of **Scottish** music and try to identify all of the **RHYTHM/TEMPO** concepts you have just studied. Several concepts may appear in one piece – for example, **4/4 time**, **strathspey**, **dotted rhythms**, **anacrusis**.

Suggested listening for Unit 8

When you have completed the brainstorm exercise, refer to the suggested listening examples for Unit 8 at www.hoddergibson. co.uk/updatesandextras or www.jm-education.com for examples of each of the above RHYTHM/TEMPO concepts.

Unit 9 National 4 TEXTURE/ STRUCTURE/FORM concepts

Canon	Theme and variation
Ternary – A B A	Cadenza
Verse and chorus	Imitation
Middle eight	

Brainstorm 9

Write down or discuss with your classmates what you know about these **TEXTURE/ STRUCTURE/FORM** concepts and think about whether you would be able to recognise each one by ear.

Activity time 12

Canon-isation

Compose a short phrase of music that can be **repeated** to create a musical **canon**. Your phrase only needs to be about four bars long and you don't have to be especially creative. You might, for example, create your four-bar **canon** phrase using just a few random notes from a **major scale**.

To test your **canon** phrase, you might play it repeatedly while other performers come in with it at staggered intervals; each beginning their phrase so that it overlaps with that of another player.

Alternatively, you can do this exercise on your own by recording your **canon** phrase repeated several times and playing over it live, or using a music sequencer.

Suggested listening for Unit 9

When you have completed the brainstorm exercise, refer to the suggested listening examples for Unit 9 at www. hoddergibson.co.uk/ updatesandextras or www.jm-education.com for examples of each of the above TEXTURE/ STRUCTURE/FORM concepts.

Unit 10 National 4 TIMBRE/DYNAMICS concepts

Brass band	Snare drum +
Wind band	Bass drum +
Violin +	Cymbals +
Cello +	Triangle +
Double bass +	Tambourine +
Harp +	Güiro
Flute +	Xylophone
Clarinet +	Glockenspiel
Saxophone	Harpsichord
Panpipes	Bass guitar
Recorder	Distortion
Trumpet +	Muted
Trombone +	Soprano, Alto, Tenor, Bass
Timpani +	Backing vocals

Brainstorm 10 !

Write down or discuss with your classmates what you know about these **TIMBRE/DYNAMICS** concepts and think about whether you would be able to recognise each one by ear.

Activity time 13

Concepts in orchestral music

Select a piece of orchestral music such as a **symphony** or a **concerto** from the **Romantic** era and see how many of the above concepts marked with a cross (+) you can identify (by ear).

Note: This is another type of listening exercise that can be repeated in other units of this chapter.

Suggested listening for Unit 10

When you have completed the brainstorm exercise, refer to the suggested listening examples for Unit 10 at www. hoddergibson.co.uk/ updatesandextras or www.jm-education.com for examples of each of the above **TIMBRE/DYNAMICS** concepts.

Concepts at work 👍

Instruments in combination

Just as colours transform into new ones when they are mixed together, so musical instruments create new sounds or **timbres** when combined. The sound of various brass instruments together, including **trombone**, **horn**, **tuba**, **cornet** and **euphonium**, make the characteristic single sound of a **brass band**; two **violins**, **viola** and **cello** combined create the sound of a **string quartet**; and the instruments in an **orchestra** offer boundless possibilities for sound combinations (see Activity time 14).

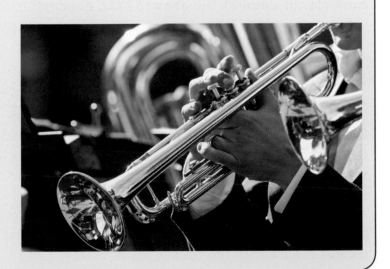

Activity time 14 ✏️

Instrumental combinations in orchestral music

Choose a few pieces of orchestral music (**symphonies**, **concertos**) from the **Classical** and **Romantic** periods and listen carefully to how instruments are combined to make many different **timbres**. Things to focus on are:

★ how instruments from the **strings** family are used to create a single **sustained** sound

★ how **woodwind** instruments such as the **flute** and **clarinet** are often combined to **harmonise** with each other

★ how the **brass** family creates drama and power in the **Romantic** music of composers such as **Mahler**, **Tchaikovsky** and **Wagner**

★ how a greater variety of **percussion** instruments are used in **Romantic** music than **Classical** to add colour and drama

National 3 musical concepts

Unit 11 National 3 STYLE concepts

Blues	Musical
Pop	Rock
Jazz	Rock 'n' roll
Latin-American	Scottish

Suggested listening for Unit 11

When you have completed the brainstorm exercise, refer to the suggested listening examples for Unit 11 at www.hoddergibson. co.uk/updatesandextras or www.jm-education.com for examples of each of the above STYLE concepts.

Brainstorm 11 ❗

Write down or discuss with your classmates what you know about these **STYLE** concepts and think about whether you would be able to recognise each one by ear.

Activity time 15 ✏️

Composing a rhythmic accompaniment

Based on the musical **STYLES** you have just looked at, select one and try composing a rhythmic accompaniment in that style. For **blues** or **rock 'n' roll** you might make up a chord progression based on **chords I, IV and V**, or create a short **pop**, **rock** or **Scottish** melody using the notes of a **pentatonic** or **major** scale. For information on these chords and scales see the musical literacy pages (17–21) and the glossary section at the end of this book.

Unit 12 National 3 MELODY/HARMONY concepts

Ascending	Question and answer
Descending	Improvisation
Step (stepwise)	Chord
Leap (leaping)	Discord
Repetition	Chord change
Sequence	

Activity time 16

Composing with concepts

Based on the **MELODY/HARMONY** concepts you have just studied, try composing short **question and answer** phrases that use **ascending** and **descending** melodies. In at least one of them include some **stepwise** and **leaping** note passages. You can do this exercise by **improvising** the phrases on an instrument, singing them, writing them on manuscript paper or using a music **sequencer**. Don't forget to save your work, as you might be able to develop these experimental phrases into a larger piece of music later (in one of the composing workshops, for example).

Activity time 17

Putting it all together

From a selection of different kinds of music, find at least one example of each of *all* the **MELODY/HARMONY** concepts (from National 5, 4 and 3) you have studied in this chapter. You can do this as a group exercise or on your own, in either case making a note of each concept as you hear it.

Note: Repeat this exercise in Units 13, 14 and 15 to ensure you understand all the concepts in each category of the National 5 course.

Suggested listening for Unit 12

When you have completed the brainstorm exercise, refer to the suggested listening examples for Unit 12 at www. hoddergibson.co.uk/ updatesandextras or www.jm-education.com for examples of each of the above MELODY/HARMONY concepts.

Concepts at work

For more information on the concepts studied in this unit, including music notation examples, see the musical literacy pages in this book and the supplementary material for the unit at **www.jm-education.com**.

Unit 13 National 3 RHYTHM/TEMPO concepts

Accent/accented	March
Beat/pulse	Reel
2, 3 and 4 beats in the bar	Waltz
On the beat/off the beat	Drum fill
Repetition	Adagio
Slower/faster	Allegro
Pause	

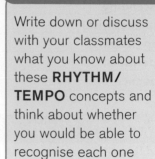

Suggested listening for Unit 13

When you have completed the brainstorm exercise, refer to the suggested listening examples for Unit 13 at www.hoddergibson. co.uk/updatesandextras or www.jm-education.com for examples of each of the above RHYTHM/TEMPO concepts.

Brainstorm 13

Write down or discuss with your classmates what you know about these **RHYTHM/TEMPO** concepts and think about whether you would be able to recognise each one by ear.

Activity time 18

Composing Scottish music

Based on the **RHYTHM/TEMPO** concepts you have just studied, compose a few musical phrases in the **STYLES** of a **march**, a **jig** and a **reel**. Include some **repetition** and a **pause**, as well as notes that are **accented** both **on the beat** and **off the beat** in at least one of your phrases. Remember, these are not whole pieces of music, just phrases that you might later develop into a larger piece. As in Activity time 16, you can compose the music by **improvising** the phrases on an instrument, singing them, writing them down freehand on manuscript paper or producing them using computer music software.

Tip maestro ⭐

When composing your new musical phrases for this unit, why not include concepts studied in previous units, such as question and answer phrases, sequence, stepwise and leaping melodies, and so on?

Unit 14 National 3 TEXTURE/ STRUCTURE/FORM concepts

Unison	Unaccompanied
Octave	Repetition
Harmony	Ostinato
Chord	Riff
Solo	Round
Accompanied	

Brainstorm 14

Write down or discuss with your classmates what you know about these **TEXTURE/ STRUCTURE/FORM** concepts and think about whether you would be able to recognise each one by ear.

Suggested listening for Unit 14

When you have completed the brainstorm exercise, refer to the suggested listening examples for Unit 14 at www.hoddergibson. co.uk/updatesandextras or www.jm-education.com for examples of each of the above **TEXTURE/STRUCTURE/FORM** concepts.

Activity time 19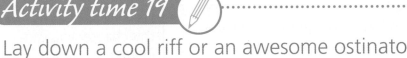

Lay down a cool riff or an awesome ostinato

Try improvising or composing a **riff** for a new piece of **blues**, **pop** or **rock** music, or an **ostinato** for a piece of instrumental music. **Repetition** is of course a feature of these concepts, but you might want to listen carefully to more examples of **riff** and **ostinato** before tackling this exercise. Later, you can try adding some **chords** and/or a **melody** to your **riff** or **ostinato**. For more advice on this, see the supplementary material for Chapter 4, Composing workshop 1: adding accompaniment parts at **www.jm-education.com**.

Concepts at work

For more information on the concepts studied in this unit, including music notation examples, see the supplementary material for the unit at **www.jm-education. com**.

Unit 15 National 3 TIMBRE/DYNAMICS concepts

Striking (Hitting) O	**Organ**
Blowing O	**Drum kit** G
Bowing O	**Steel band**
Strumming G	**Scottish dance band**
Plucking G	**Folk group**
Accordion S	**Voice** G
Fiddle S	**Choir**
Bagpipes S	**Staccato** O
Acoustic guitar S	**Legato** O
Electric guitar G	**Orchestra (strings, brass, woodwind and percussion – tuned and untuned)**
Piano S	

Brainstorm 15

Write down or discuss with your classmates what you know about these **TIMBRE/ DYNAMICS** concepts and think about whether you would be able to recognise each one by ear.

Suggested listening for Unit 15

When you have completed the brainstorm exercise, refer to the suggested listening examples for Unit 15 at www.hoddergibson. co.uk/updatesandextras or www.jm-education.com for examples of each of the above **TIMBRE/DYNAMICS** concepts.

Activity time 20

O, G and S

Next to some of the concepts in the list on page 15 you will notice the letters 'O', 'G' and 'S'. These refer to **orchestral**, **group** and **Scottish**, and are there to help you in this exercise, which requires you to find an example of a concept specifically from pieces of **orchestral** music, a **group** of your choice (rock, folk, pop etc.) and **Scottish** music.

So, '**Blowing O**' means you have to identify the concept **blowing** in a piece of **orchestral** music, '**Strumming G**' asks you to find an example of **strumming** performed in a **group**, and '**Acoustic guitar S**' requires you to find a piece of **Scottish** music that uses an **acoustic guitar**. Each of the three musical styles has **five** concepts for you to identify.

For this exercise you should find your own examples. Do not use those given in the list of Suggested listening for this unit.

Concepts at work

Every time you hear a piece of music from now on – on the TV or radio, at the supermarket or on your computer – listen carefully and see how many of the concepts you have studied in this chapter you can identify. Now that you have learned them, listen out to hear those concepts at work.

This chapter covers the musical literacy (or music theory) requirements for National 5, National 4 and National 3. Musical literacy is the term given to the study of notes, terms and symbols used in music notation – the 'language' of music. Even a basic knowledge of this language will increase your understanding (and enjoyment) of all types of music, and prepare you for the final National 5 Listening test, which contains questions on musical literacy (see question 3 of the specimen listening test question paper on page 24).

The literacy concepts for each level are clearly set out in music notation for quick and easy reference.

National 3 musical literacy

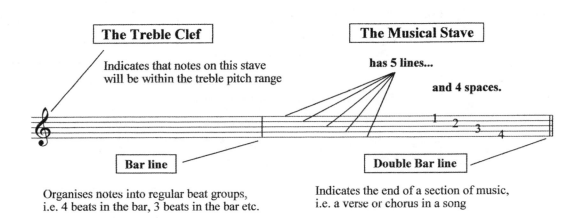

The Treble Clef
Indicates that notes on this stave will be within the treble pitch range

The Musical Stave
has 5 lines...
and 4 spaces.

Bar line
Organises notes into regular beat groups, i.e. 4 beats in the bar, 3 beats in the bar etc.

Double Bar line
Indicates the end of a section of music, i.e. a verse or chorus in a song

---

Note Values

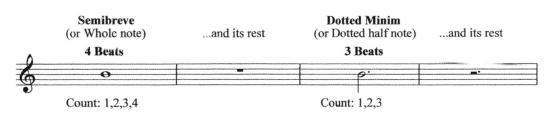

Semibreve (or Whole note) ...and its rest   Dotted Minim (or Dotted half note) ...and its rest
4 Beats   3 Beats
Count: 1,2,3,4   Count: 1,2,3

Minim (or Half note) ...and its rest   Crotchet (or Quarter note) ...and its rest
2 Beats   1 Beat
Count: 1,2   Count: 1

Steps and Repetition

Notes moving by Step   Repetition (of notes in previous bar)

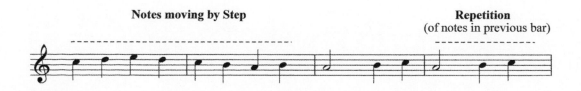

Dynamics

f - **forte** (loud)   ***p*** - **piano** (quiet)

cresc. ———————————   **crescendo - gradually louder**   *dim.* ———————————   **diminuendo - gradually quieter**

National 4 musical literacy

Notes on the Treble Clef Stave

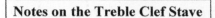

C   D   E   F   G   A   B   C   D   E   F   G   A

Sequences and Repeat Signs

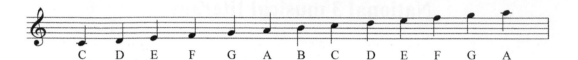

Repeat sign   Repeat sign

Bar 1   Sequences of bar 1: (Bar 1 repeated at lower and higher pitches)

lower pitch   higher pitch   higher pitch

Repeat the music between the repeat signs

Dynamics

mf - **mezzo forte** (moderately loud)   ***mp*** - **mezzo piano** (moderately quiet)

Quavers (eighth notes)

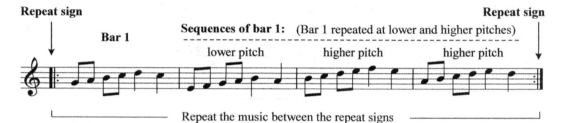

single quaver   its rest   paired quavers   quavers can also be grouped in fours

Some common quaver groupings

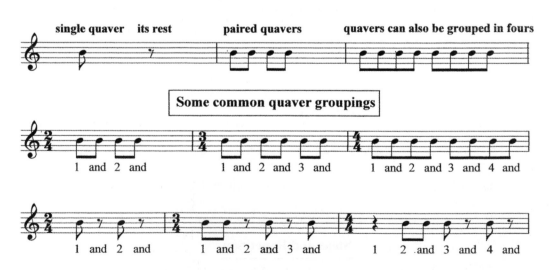

1 and 2 and   1 and 2 and 3 and   1 and 2 and 3 and 4 and

1 and 2 and   1 and 2 and 3 and   1   2 and 3 and 4 and

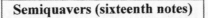

Semiquavers (sixteenth notes)

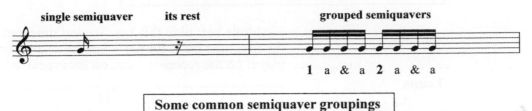

single semiquaver　　　its rest　　　　　　　grouped semiquavers

1　a　&　a　2　a　&　a

Some common semiquaver groupings

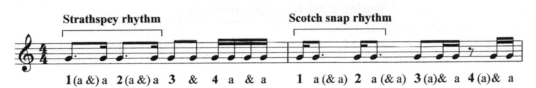

1　a　&　a　2　a　& (a)　　　1 (a) & a　2　a　& (a)　3　(a) & (a)　4

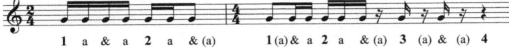

Strathspey rhythm　　　　　　　Scotch snap rhythm

1 (a &) a　2 (a &) a　3　&　4　a　& a　　　1　a (& a)　2　a (& a)　3 (a) & a　4 (a) & a

Note: beats displayed in brackets indicate semiquaver beats which are counted but not played

National 5 musical literacy

Tones and Semitones

The 'natural' notes in music (A B C D E F G - no sharps or flats used) have two naturally occurring **semitones** between the notes **B** and **C**, and the notes **E** and **F**. The other notes are a **tone** apart.

All adjacent keys on a piano or keyboard are a semitone apart. Tones are two keys apart. **Two semitones** make a **tone**.

The **C major** scale

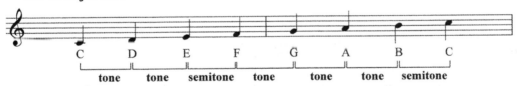

C　　D　　E　　F　　G　　A　　B　　C

tone　　tone　　semitone　　tone　　tone　　tone　　semitone

To maintain the above order of tones and semitones in other scales, **accidentals** have to be used. These are shown at the start in **key signatures** (see *Scales and Key Signatures*).

Accidentals

An accidental is a symbol, placed in front of a note, which alters the pitch of that note.

There are three main kinds: the **SHARP** ♯   the **FLAT** ♭   and the **NATURAL** ♮

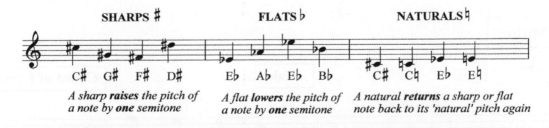

SHARPS ♯　　　　　　　FLATS ♭　　　　　　　NATURALS ♮

C♯　G♯　F♯　D♯　　　E♭　A♭　E♭　B♭　　　C♯　C♮　E♭　E♮

*A sharp **raises** the pitch of a note by **one** semitone*　*A flat **lowers** the pitch of a note by **one** semitone*　*A natural **returns** a sharp or flat note back to its 'natural' pitch again*

IMPORTANT RULE: A note which has been made sharp or flat will stay that way until the next bar, where it returns to its 'natural' pitch. The sharp or flat sign will only be used ONCE but it will apply for the whole bar, unless a natural is used to cancel it.

Leaps & First and Second Time Bars

First time bar: play this bar the first time only; do not play it on the repeat

Second time bar: play this bar the second time, on the repeat

Leaps

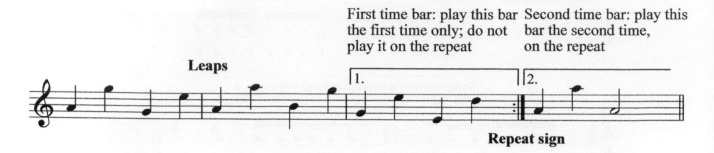

Repeat sign

Scales and Key Signatures

Key: C Major

Key signature (no sharps or flats)

Scale

Chord of C major

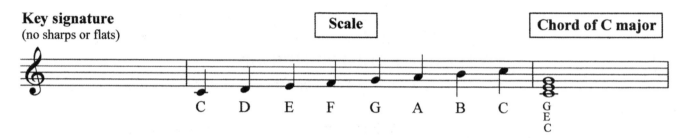

C D E F G A B C

G
E
C

Key: G Major

Key signature (one sharp: F#)

Scale

Chord of G major

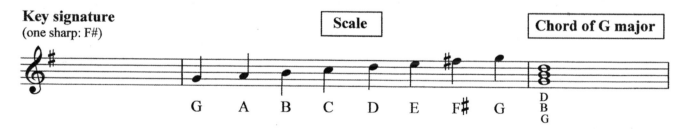

G A B C D E F# G

D
B
G

Key: F Major

Key signature (one flat: B♭)

Scale

Chord of F major

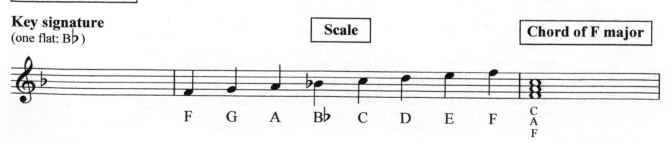

F G A B♭ C D E F

C
A
F

Key: A Minor

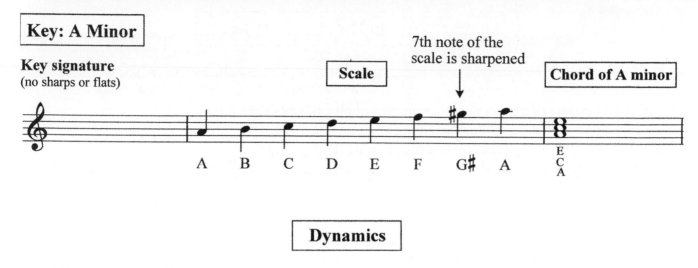

Key signature
(no sharps or flats)

Scale

7th note of the
scale is sharpened

Chord of A minor

A B C D E F G♯ A

E
C
A

Dynamics

ff - **fortissimo** (very loud)   *pp* - **pianissimo** (very quiet)

sfz - **sforzando** (suddenly loud)

Dotted Rhythms

When a dot appears **after** a note it adds on *half* the value of that note again

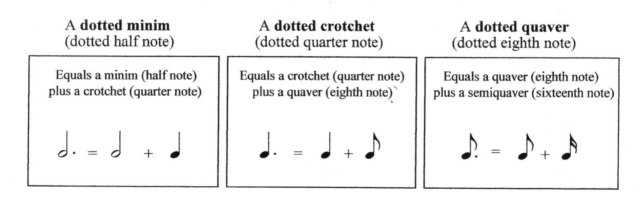

A dotted minim
(dotted half note)

Equals a minim (half note)
plus a crotchet (quarter note)

A dotted crotchet
(dotted quarter note)

Equals a crotchet (quarter note)
plus a quaver (eighth note)

A dotted quaver
(dotted eighth note)

Equals a quaver (eighth note)
plus a semiquaver (sixteenth note)

This is how these rhythms are counted (brackets show beats on which no notes are played):

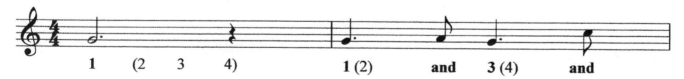

1   (2   3   4)   1 (2)   and   3 (4)   and

These **dotted rhythms** are common in **Scottish** music, especially **Strathspeys**

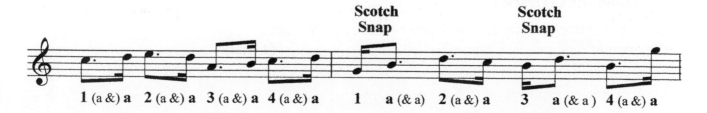

Scotch
Snap

Scotch
Snap

1 (a &) a   2 (a &) a   3 (a &) a   4 (a &) a   1   a (& a)   2 (a &) a   3   a (& a)   4 (a &) a

This chapter consists of a specimen listening test question paper similar to the one you will sit in the exam at the end of your National 5 Music course. Before attempting it you should have first worked through Chapters 1 and 2, since both of these chapters contain essential material to prepare you for the listening test itself.

It is also important that you take the test in one sitting, following the instructions of each question very carefully, just as you would in the actual exam. This will allow you to make an accurate assessment of your readiness to sit the exam.

With these points in mind, it is recommended that you attempt the listening test in this chapter towards the end of your course.

Either write your answers in this book (if it is your own copy) or on a separate sheet of paper.

Activity time 21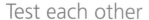

Test each other

When you have completed this chapter, you and a few of your study partners or classmates could prepare a listening test for each other, based on the eight question types in this specimen paper. Before you put yourselves to the test, however, make sure that every 'examiner' has made a note of the correct answers.

Specimen listening test

Question 1

This question is about different **styles** of music.

🔊 **Listen Up: CD track 1**

a) Listen to CD track 1 and tick **one** box to describe what you hear. **(1 mark)**

☐ Pop
☐ Gospel
☐ Musical
☐ Rock 'n' roll

🔊 **Listen Up: CD track 1**

b) Listen to CD track 1 again and write **one** concept that describes the texture. **(1 mark)**

🔊 **Listen Up: CD track 2**

c) Listen to a different piece of music on CD track 2 and tick **one** box to describe what you hear. **(1 mark)**
   ☐ Symphony
   ☐ Concerto
   ☐ Minimalist
   ☐ Gaelic psalm

🔊 **Listen Up: CD track 2**

d) Listen to CD track 2 again and name the ornament played by the solo instrument near the end of the track. **(1 mark)**

_____

🔊 **Listen Up: CD track 3**

e) Listen to a new excerpt of music on CD track 3 and tick **one** box to describe what you hear. **(1 mark)**
   ☐ Symphony
   ☐ Baroque
   ☐ Concerto
   ☐ Minimalism

🔊 **Listen Up: CD track 3**

f) Listen to the same excerpt again and write the Italian term that describes the string playing technique. **(1 mark)**

_____

Total marks Question 1: (6) ☐

Question 2

In this question you will listen to an excerpt of instrumental music.

A guide to the music has been laid out on page 24. You will see that further information is required and you should insert this in each of the four areas.

Give yourself 1 minute to read through the question before listening to CD track 4.

You can listen to the music **three** times, allowing no more than 30 seconds between playings.

A voice will help guide you through the music.

🔊 **Listen Up: CD track 4**

Following the instructions above, listen to CD track 4 and insert your answers on the diagram on page 24. **(4 marks)**

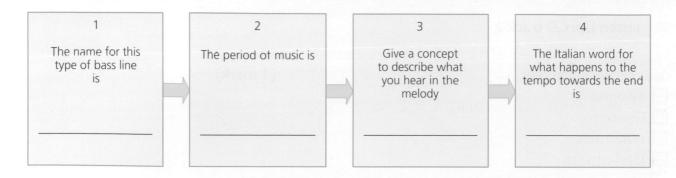

1	2	3	4
The name for this type of bass line is	The period of music is	Give a concept to describe what you hear in the melody	The Italian word for what happens to the tempo towards the end is

Total marks Question 2: (4) ☐

Question 3

You now have to answer questions relating to the music printed below.

🔊 **Listen Up: CD track 5**

Listen to CD track 5 and follow the music. Do not write anything during this first listening. You should listen to the track another **three** times, allowing no more than 30 seconds between playings. After the final playing allow 2 minutes to complete your answers.

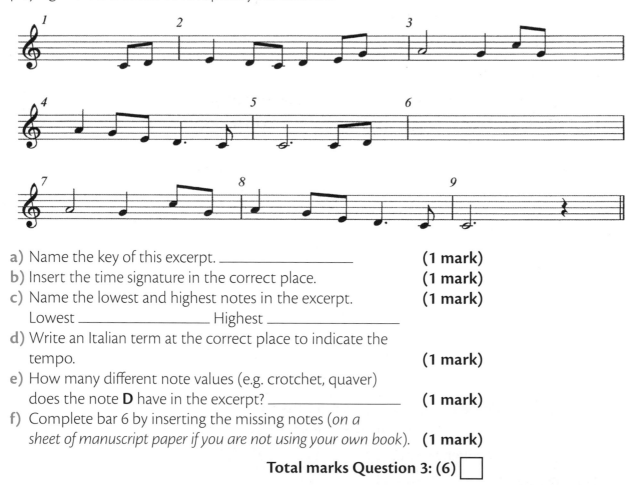

a) Name the key of this excerpt. _____ **(1 mark)**
b) Insert the time signature in the correct place. **(1 mark)**
c) Name the lowest and highest notes in the excerpt. **(1 mark)**
   Lowest _____ Highest _____
d) Write an Italian term at the correct place to indicate the tempo. **(1 mark)**
e) How many different note values (e.g. crotchet, quaver) does the note **D** have in the excerpt? _____ **(1 mark)**
f) Complete bar 6 by inserting the missing notes (*on a sheet of manuscript paper if you are not using your own book*). **(1 mark)**

Total marks Question 3: (6) ☐

Question 4

This question features **vocal** music.

🔊 **Listen Up: CD track 6**

a) Listen to CD track 6 and tick **one** box to describe what you hear. **(1 mark)**

- ☐ Jazz
- ☐ Mouth music
- ☐ Swing
- ☐ Aria

🔊 **Listen Up: CD track 7**

b) Listen to CD track 7 and name the style. **(1 mark)**

_____

🔊 **Listen Up: CD track 8**

c) Listen to CD track 8 and tick **one** box to describe what you hear. **(1 mark)**

- ☐ Soprano
- ☐ Mezzo-soprano
- ☐ Alto
- ☐ Tenor

🔊 **Listen Up: CD track 9**

d) Listen to CD track 9 and tick **one** box to identify the chord sequence heard in this song. Listen to the track no more than **twice**, with a pause of up to 10 seconds between playings.

The music is in the key of G major. **(1 mark)**

☐
I	IV	V	VI
G	C	D	Em

☐
I	VI	IV	V
G	Em	C	D

☐
I	V	VI	IV
G	D	Em	C

🔊 **Listen Up: CD track 10**

e) Listen to CD track 10 and tick **two** boxes to describe features of the music. **(2 marks)**

- ☐ Syllabic
- ☐ Backing vocals
- ☐ Homophonic
- ☐ Descant
- ☐ Polyphonic

🔊 **Listen Up: CD track 11**

f) Listen to more music from the same piece on CD track 11 and tick **one** box to describe what you hear. **(1 mark)**
- ☐ Rubato
- ☐ Accelerando
- ☐ Syncopation
- ☐ Cross rhythms

🔊 **Listen Up: CD track 11**

g) Listen to CD track 11 again and name the percussion instrument playing. **(1 mark)**

_____

Total marks Question 4: (8) ☐

Question 5

In this question you will listen to an excerpt of a Scottish dance **three** times.

Tick **one** answer only in each of the four sections:

Solo instrument, Accompanying instrument, Scottish dance, Tempo

Take 30 seconds to read the question before hearing the excerpt.

🔊 **Listen Up: CD track 12**

Listen to CD track 12 and tick **one** answer in each of the four sections. Listen to the track no more than **three times**, with a pause of up to 10 seconds between playings. **(4 marks)**

		Tick	
Solo instrument	Flute		Tick one box from this section
	Bagpipes		
	Accordion		
Accompanying instrument	Snare drum		Tick one box from this section
	Clàrsach		
	Bodhrán		
Scottish dance	Waltz		Tick one box from this section
	Reel		
	Strathspey		
Tempo	Andante		Tick one box from this section
	Adagio		
	Allegro		

Total marks Question 5: (4) ☐

Question 6

In this question you are asked to describe the music that you hear by inserting the appropriate concepts in the text below.

Give yourself no more than 20 seconds to read through the question.

🔊 **Listen Up: CD track 13**

Listen to CD track 13 no more than **twice**, allowing a pause of 10 seconds between playings, and insert the concepts in the text below.　　**(3 marks)**

There are _____ beats in each bar.

A small group of instruments from the _____ family join in playing the melody.

The excerpt is in _____ form.

Total marks Question 6: (3) ☐

Question 7

This question features **instrumental** music.

🔊 **Listen Up: CD track 14**

a) As you listen to CD track 14:
　i) tick **one** box to describe the style of music　　　　**(1 mark)**
　ii) give a reason to support your answer　　　　　　　**(1 mark)**

　☐ Jazz
　☐ African
　☐ Indian
　☐ Latin-American

Reason _____

🔊 **Listen Up: CD track 15**

b) As you listen to a different excerpt on CD track 15:
　i) tick **one** box to describe the style of music　　　　**(1 mark)**
　ii) give a reason to support your answer　　　　　　　**(1 mark)**

　☐ Baroque
　☐ Classical
　☐ Romantic
　☐ Cadenza

Reason _____

Total marks Question 7: (4) ☐

Question 8

🔊 **Listen Up: CD track 16**

As you listen to CD track 16, write about the prominent features of the music. Listen to the track no more than **three** times and afterwards give yourself 2 minutes to complete your final answer.

In your answer, comment on at least **three** of the following:

- Rhythm/tempo
- Melody/harmony
- Instruments/voices
- Dynamics

You can use the table below for rough working, but your final answer must be written on the lines below FINAL ANSWER. **(5 marks)**

ROUGH WORK

Rhythm/tempo	
Melody/harmony	
Instruments/voices	
Dynamics	

FINAL ANSWER

_____

_____

_____

_____

_____

_____

_____

Total marks Question

Note: Additional material for this chapter, including two complete workshops (**Composing a dance track using a MIDI sequencer** and **Analysing a modern song**) can be found on the website **www.jm-education.com**.

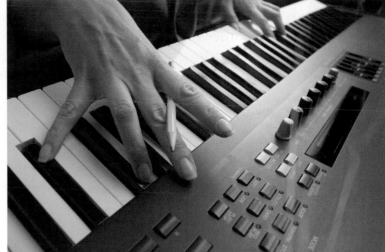

The composing assignment draws on students' skills, knowledge and understanding of music composition. Its purpose is to allow students to demonstrate their skills in the use of at least three of the following:
- melody
- harmony
- rhythm
- timbre
- structure

when creating their piece of music. Candidates show their understanding of these different elements through the creative and effective development of a range of musical ideas.

The following items must be included:
- an audio recording
- a score or performance plan
- a composing review (see page 57).

This chapter demonstrates various step-by-step composing techniques in two contrasting workshops. The purpose of the step-by-step approach is to highlight the techniques that can be used to generate whole pieces of structured music from basic ideas.

In workshop 1 we will compose a piece of instrumental music starting with just a few notes, while in workshop 2 we examine techniques for setting words to music (song writing).

These workshops use a broad range of musical concepts and literacy terms so it will make things easier if you have already worked through Chapters 1 and 2.

Composing workshop 1: Composing a short instrumental piece

We are now going to compose a complete piece of instrumental music. It doesn't matter whether or not you have composed any music before since we will be going through everything one step at a time. Even if you are a bit more experienced, however, you should still work through each step in sequence. Doing so will give you the chance to try some of the techniques often used by professional composers. Most of these techniques can also be applied to song writing and will therefore be helpful in workshop 2 as well.

Where do I begin?

There are a few ways in which we might approach composing a new piece of music. Often it starts with the composer playing around (**improvising**) with notes on a musical instrument until some good ideas present themselves. But how do you develop those first ideas, or turn that one great *phrase* of music into a great *piece* of music? And what if you don't come up with anything? Is it possible to sit down and compose something good from scratch?

Yes! Using the techniques in this workshop you will see that it is not only possible but fairly simple to generate ideas and musical phrases from nothing other than some notes in a musical scale, and then develop these into a well-structured piece of music.

Finding inspiration

Much like a story, you can write a piece of music about almost anything: your feelings about someone or something, a place, a major sporting event, something scary or something peaceful. It can either be a song, or an instrumental piece that expresses the subject through musical **keys**, **dynamics**, **tempo** and **rhythm** rather than words.

Unlike a written story, however, music has the added advantage that it doesn't *have* to be about anything in particular. You can compose a piece and simply call it 'study', or use the **tempo** as the title – for example, **allegro**, **andante** or **adagio**. Famous composers have done this over the centuries so you would be in very distinguished company.

Musical structure or form

Most types of music have a structure which creates a sense of 'order' that is satisfying to hear. Songs are usually made up of **verses** and a **chorus**, perhaps also with a **middle 8** (or **bridge** passage) and a short instrumental interlude. Common structures for instrumental music include **binary**, **ternary**, **rondo**, **canon** and **fugue**.

Short instrumental pieces or 'miniatures' often have a **binary** or **ternary**
structure. Music that has no repetitive structure, or that seems spontaneous, is called **through-composed**.

Step 1: the structure plan

As we know, it is possible to begin a new composition by **improvising** to see if a piece 'grows'. However, there are several advantages to starting out with a plan:

Tip maestro

Learn by observing and listening ...

Writers read books by other authors, artists visit galleries to look at the work of other artists, and composers listen to a lot of music by other composers. This activity is like feeding the mind with examples and inspiration that it will process into new ideas of its own.

*No serious, self-respecting composer or artist would steal from someone else's work, but they all allow themselves to be **influenced** by the work of others. Listening to music and studying printed music notation — especially music in the style in which you intend to compose — will increase your understanding and give you ideas for a composition. So a good way to start a new piece of music might be to consider the kind of music you like most and then try writing something in the same style. That way you are likely to stay more motivated as you work through the piece, not to mention being better acquainted with the musical concepts required.*

- It will make the composing process more straightforward.
- You are far less likely to become stuck for ideas on how to complete your composition.
- Your finished piece will be well-structured and sound accomplished.
- It will give you confidence to develop the piece into a much larger composition if you want.
- You can see the whole piece as a 'sketch' or a 'map' from the very beginning. This makes it easier to see where you might put all your musical ideas.

For the composition in this workshop I have chosen a **ternary** structure. This is a common structure for short instrumental compositions, and has been used in **Baroque** and **Classical** music and especially in the instrumental 'miniatures' of the **Romantic** era.

Ternary form has three sections, which we can call **A B A**. It is a nicely symmetrical structure in which the first 'A' section can be regarded as the **beginning**, 'B' the contrasting **middle** section, and then the **repeat** of the 'A' section as the **end** of the piece.

I have decided to make each section eight bars long (two four-bar phrases), meaning that the whole piece will be 24 bars in length. This is a sort of 'first draft' that I can extend later if I want – perhaps by **repeating** one or more of the **sections** (possibly with some **variation** added), or by including a **coda** at the end. I might even choose to extend the **ternary** structure (**A B A**) into a **rondo** by adding another contrasting section (C), followed by a **repeat** of the A section, to make an **A B A C A** structure.

Mapping the structure

You can start with a table (like the one below) or by mapping out 24 empty bars on a piece of music manuscript, and writing in the main sections (see example on page 32). This will give you a useful visual reference of your entire piece even before you compose a single note.

Here is my table showing the main structural events:

A Section	B Section	A Section repeat
Bars 1–8 (two four-bar phrases)	Bars 9–16 (two four-bar phrases)	Bars 17–24 (two four-bar phrases)
Main musical ideas	**Contrast (key change)** **New musical ideas**	**Main musical ideas** **repeated with variation**

At this point we could sit down with a musical instrument and start **improvising** – experimenting with notes and phrases until we come up with something that can be developed into an eight-bar A section. However, I want to introduce you to useful composing techniques, so instead I'm going to show you another helpful step towards creating a good structure.

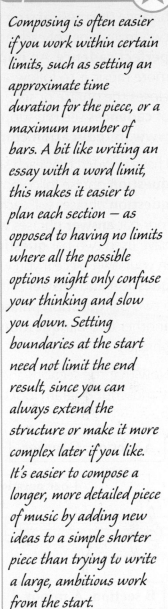

Tip maestro

Composing is often easier if you work within certain limits, such as setting an approximate time duration for the piece, or a maximum number of bars. A bit like writing an essay with a word limit, this makes it easier to plan each section – as opposed to having no limits where all the possible options might only confuse your thinking and slow you down. Setting boundaries at the start need not limit the end result, since you can always extend the structure or make it more complex later if you like. It's easier to compose a longer, more detailed piece of music by adding new ideas to a simple shorter piece than trying to write a large, ambitious work from the start.

Phrases and cadences

Choosing the **cadence** points at this early stage in our piece will balance the musical structure and make it sound 'right' to the ear. The two main types of cadence are the **imperfect cadence** and the **perfect cadence**. An **imperfect cadence** is like a comma, suggesting more music is to follow, and a **perfect cadence** is like a 'full stop' that closes the phrase or section. For more information on the construction of **cadences** see the supplementary material for this chapter at **www.jm-education.com**.

I have decided that each section of my piece will begin with a four-bar **question** phrase followed by a four-bar **answer** phrase. The four-bar **question** phrases will each end with an **imperfect cadence**, and the four-bar **answer** phrases with a **perfect cadence**. (I could just as easily have used two-bar **question and answer** phrases, and you can do this in your own piece if you wish, but you will need to have two sets of **question and answer** phrases to make the eight-bar total. For example: a two-bar **question** phrase followed by a two-bar **answer** phrase, then another two-bar **question** phrase followed by a second two-bar **answer** phrase.)

Now that the sections and **cadences** have been planned out, my manuscript diagram looks like this:

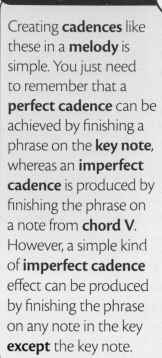

Concepts at work

Creating **cadences** like these in a **melody** is simple. You just need to remember that a **perfect cadence** can be achieved by finishing a phrase on the **key note**, whereas an **imperfect cadence** is produced by finishing the phrase on a note from **chord V**. However, a simple kind of **imperfect cadence** effect can be produced by finishing the phrase on any note in the key **except** the key note.

Drawing the diagram and identifying the location of the **cadences** beforehand guarantees that the piece will have a good structure even before we add a single note. It already has a symmetry, which will make it sound balanced and flowing.

Activity time 22

Get a bit of structure

Make a structure plan for your own piece now. You can do this as a diagram or, if you prefer, using music manuscript. You don't have to choose the same key as I did (**C major**) since the techniques we will be using can be applied to any key, but if you are completely new to composing it might be better to do so as you will then be able to follow my steps more easily. Better still, why not use my guidelines to write your first instrumental piece then compose another in a different key?

Step 2: thinking about musical concepts

I'm now going to make a list of some musical concepts I might use in my piece. Once I have this list I can keep referring to it as I compose.

Possible melody concepts	Possible rhythm/tempo concepts
Question and answer phrases	**Accents**
Ascending/descending melody	**Pause**
Stepwise/leaping melody	**Syncopation**
Repetition	**Scotch snap**
Sequence	**Anacrusis**
Key change	**Dotted rhythms**
Variation	**Accelerando (accel.)**
Chromatic notes	**Rallentando (rall.)**
Passing notes	

Tip maestro

Think of musical concepts like colours on an artist's palette. The more colours there are the more options are available to the artist for his or her painting. So the more musical concepts the musician is aware of, the more scope there is for an interesting piece of music.

Making the music

Step 3: the melody — composing the first four-bar 'question' phrase

The first step in composing the **melody** is to choose a **key**, since this will give us a musical **scale** from which we can choose notes to develop our first ideas. You will remember that I have chosen the key of **C major**. The scale notes in this key are C, D, E, F, G, A, B. The available chords are: **C major**, **D minor**, **E minor**, **F major**, **G major**, **A minor** and **B diminished**. (For more information on **keys** and **chords** refer to **Scales and key signatures**, page 20, and the supplementary material for this chapter at **www.jm-education.com**.)

To create some ideas for a possible **melody**, we could improvise using these notes and **chords**, making a note of which bits we like best, and of course experimenting with other concepts such as **chromatic notes**, **grace notes**, **trills**, **glissando** and so on. (This would also be a good time to refer to the list of possible **MELODY** and **RHYTHM/TEMPO** concepts above.) Using the notes of the **C major** scale, here is what I came up with for my first four-bar **question** phrase. (For a detailed, bar-by-bar analysis of this phrase, see the supplementary material for this workshop at **www.jm-education.com**.)

Tip maestro

*Sometimes composers and songwriters come up with a progression of **chords** first, to which they then write a **melody**.*

The A section (bars 1–4: the question phrase)

A Section (C major)

First 4-bar phrase (bars 1-4)

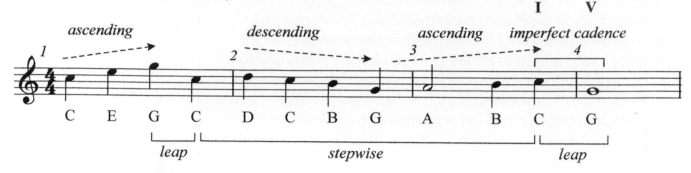

Concepts used: ascending and **descending** melody; **stepwise** melody and **leaps**; **imperfect cadence**.

Summary: Most of this phrase moves by **step**. Its **ascending** and **descending** note patterns create a wave-like shape.

This opening phrase is simple, but it has a pleasing sound – which is the important thing. What's more, I already have enough material in these four bars to generate lots of new ideas for the rest of the piece.

Activity time 23

The A section question phrase

Now compose an opening four-bar **question** phrase for your own piece, remembering the processes and concepts I used. Don't forget to end the phrase with an **imperfect cadence**.

Through its **key** and the concepts it uses, my first four-bar phrase has already set a style and mood for the whole piece. I can of course **repeat** some or all of this phrase later (in a **ternary** structure the whole A section is usually repeated), but with the help of some clever **variation and development techniques** I can also turn it into several new phrases – without having to think up a single new bar of music.

Concepts at work

Variation and development techniques

Here are some techniques that can be used to develop new music from a phrase you have already composed. You will see how I use them throughout this workshop, and you can refer to this page as you compose each new phrase of your own piece.

★ Experiment with how a phrase sounds when played **backwards**, or when the music is turned **upside down**. You can even try playing it **upside down and backwards**. (See supplementary material at **www.jm-education.com** for more information on this.)

⇨

Tip maestro ★

Remember: these techniques of development are not an alternative to being musically creative, but a way of giving yourself fresh ideas and generating new music that you might not have thought of otherwise. (They are one reason why experienced composers can write good music fairly quickly.) However, music is an art, not a structural science, so always listen carefully to your composition as it develops and trust your instincts. If it doesn't sound good to you, try something different.

⇨
★ **Repeat part** of a bar or phrase in another, new phrase.
★ **Repeat** a bar or phrase but **vary** it slightly by making small **note** or **rhythm** changes, or adding **passing notes** where possible (these give the music more **rhythm**/movement).
★ **Repeat** the **notes** of a previous bar or phrase but use a different **rhythm**.
★ **Repeat** the **rhythm** of a previous bar or phrase but use different **notes**.
★ Use the **notes** of a **chord** to create a bar or several bars of music.
★ Use **sequence**.
★ **Repeat** a phrase but increase or decrease the note values. For example, **crotchets** (**quarter notes**) could be made twice as long to become **minims** (**half notes**), or half as long to become **quavers** (**eighth notes**).

Step 4: the A section (bars 5–8: the answer phrase)

In order to complete the A section I now need to compose the **answer** phrase to bars 1–4, and end it with a **perfect cadence**. To begin, I played bars 1–4 over a few times to see if I could 'hear' in my head a phrase that naturally responded to the **question** phrase. I felt that the notes at the start of the new phrase should probably be **ascending**. To make a strong **perfect cadence** at the end I would also have to make the last note the key note, **C**.

Here is the result:

A Section

Second 4-bar phrase (bars 5-8)

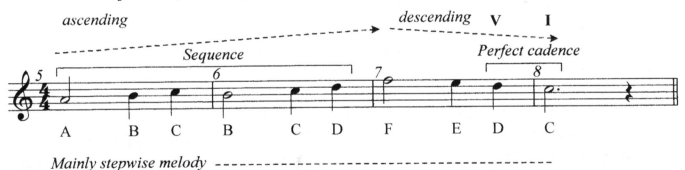

Concepts used: ascending and **descending** melody, **sequence**, **stepwise** melody, **perfect cadence**.

Summary: Another mainly **stepwise** phrase with a very clear **ascending** melody that **descends** towards the **perfect cadence** at the end.

Note:

1 This four-bar **answer** phrase has an **ascending-descending** shape.

2 Bars 5, 6 and 7 use the same **rhythm**.

For a bar-by-bar analysis see **www.jm-education.com**.

🔊 **Listen Up: CD track 17**

Listen to the four-bar **question and answer** phrases on CD track 17 that make my eight-bar A section and follow the music below.

A Section (bars 1-8)

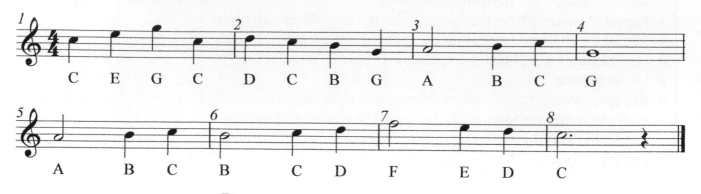

Bars 1-4: C E G C | D C B G | A B C G |
A B C B | C D F | E D C

Activity time 24 ✏️

The A section answer phrase

When you have carefully studied/listened to the eight bars of my A section – noting how everything was put together – compose an **answer** phrase to complete your own A section. Remember to use a **perfect cadence** to close the section.

Step 5: the B section (bars 9–12: the question phrase)

This section is about **contrast**. To achieve this, I'm going to change key. Common **key changes** or **modulations** are linked to **chords IV**, **V** and **VI**. In my key of **C major**, typical **key modulations** would therefore be to **F major** (chord IV), **G major** (chord V) or **A minor** (chord VI, the *relative minor key**). I'm going with **A minor** since the other two keys are **major**. Using a **minor** key will provide a greater sense of contrast, especially in a short piece of music like this.

> *A **relative minor key** gets its name from the fact that it has the same **key signature** as one other **major key**, and is therefore said to be related to that key. Every **major key** has a **relative minor key** and vice versa (see supplementary material at **www.jm-education.com**).

Having changed key I now have a new **scale** and set of **chords**. The **seventh** note of a **minor** scale is normally raised by a **semitone** (sharpened) – so the notes of the **A minor scale** are: **A, B, C, D, E, F** and **G#**. (Any G notes I use in the melody from now on will have to be sharpened until I change key again.) The main **chords** in **A minor** are: **A minor** (chord I), **D minor** (chord IV), **E major** (chord V) and **F major** (chord VI).

In addition to the **key change**, I also wanted to include some new concepts in the piece, so I referred back to the concept list I made earlier (page 33).

With all this information helping to guide me, it didn't take long to compose the next four bars of my piece.

B Section (A minor)

First 4-bar phrase (bars 9-12)

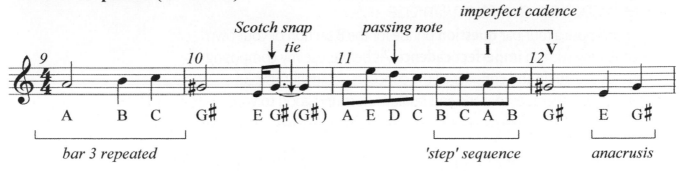

Scotch snap   *passing note*   *imperfect cadence*

A   B   C   G♯   E G♯ (G♯)   A E D C   B C A B   G♯   E G♯

bar 3 repeated   *'step' sequence*   *anacrusis*

Concepts used: key change, repetition, Scotch snap, passing note, 'step' sequence, imperfect cadence, anacrusis.

Summary: This phrase is a little more active than the music of the A section, and uses a **Scotch snap** and **quavers** (**eighth notes**) for the first time. Most of the melody was influenced by the **chords** of **A minor** (**chord I**

in the new key of **A minor**) and **E major** (**chord V**).

Note: A **tie** is used in bar 10. A **tie** is a line that joins together ('ties') the time value of two notes of the **same** pitch. The second note is not played but its duration is added onto the first.

For a bar-by-bar analysis see **www.jm-education.com**.

Concepts at work 👍

'Step' sequence

As its name implies, a 'step' **sequence** moves by step. This particular kind of **sequence** has an unmistakable pattern. Each note is followed by another that is either a step higher or a step lower.

Consider the following two bars of music:

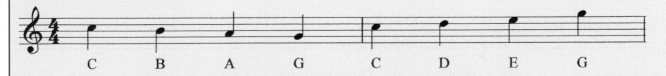

C   B   A   G   C   D   E   G

We can develop this phrase by adding a 'step' **sequence**. In the example below, the arrows pointing upwards indicate the added notes that move a step **higher** than the original notes, and the arrows pointing downwards those that go a step **lower**. The original notes are **circled**.

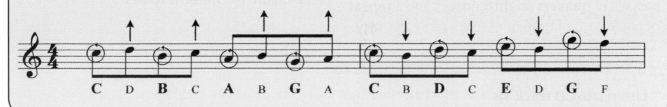

C D **B** c **A** b **G** a   **C** b **D** c **E** d **G** f

Activity time 25

The B section question phrase

Now compose a four-bar **question** phrase for the B section of your own piece, ending with an **imperfect cadence**. As before, use my composing methods as a guide and consider all the concepts you might use. Be creative, but remember that the end result must sound good to you.

Step 6: the B section (bars 13–16: the answer phrase)

This phrase will complete the B section, ending with a **perfect cadence**. It will also be the last piece of original **melody** I need to compose since everything that follows will be the product of **repetition** or **variation** techniques.

Even though the B section is in the key of **A minor**, I'm going to end it in **C major**, creating a **modulation** back to the original key to anticipate the **repeat** of the A section. I will therefore end the phrase with the notes **G** (from **G major**, **chord V** in **C major**), and **C** (from **C major**, **chord I**), thereby making a **V–I perfect cadence** in **C major**. Now all I have to do is work out some notes that follow on naturally from the last phrase (bars 9–12).

Tip maestro

Rests *can be used very effectively to shape musical phrases because they create natural pauses – as though the music is 'taking a breath' before resuming with the next phrase.*

B Section (A minor)

Second 4-bar phrase (bars 13-16)

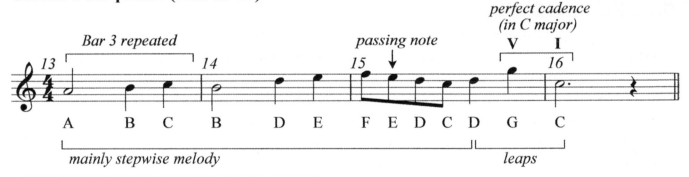

Concepts used: repetition, **stepwise** melody, **passing note**, **leaps**, **perfect cadence**.

Summary: Although a little less active than the previous phrase (bars 9–12), this one still has a passage of **quavers** (**eighth notes**), and a **repeat** of bar 3. Both of these preserve a sense of **unity** with the rest of the piece so far. The **perfect cadence** in **C major** will return us smoothly into the A section **repeat**, while the **crotchet** (**quarter note**) **rest** at the end creates a brief pause before the music resumes.

For a bar-by-bar analysis see **www.jm-education.com**.

🔊 **Listen Up: CD track 18**

On page 39 is the basic first draft of my piece, complete with a **repeat** of the A section (no **variation** added yet). Follow the music as you listen to CD track 18. Notice that, thanks to my early planning of phrase lengths and **cadences**, it is well-structured and sounds balanced.

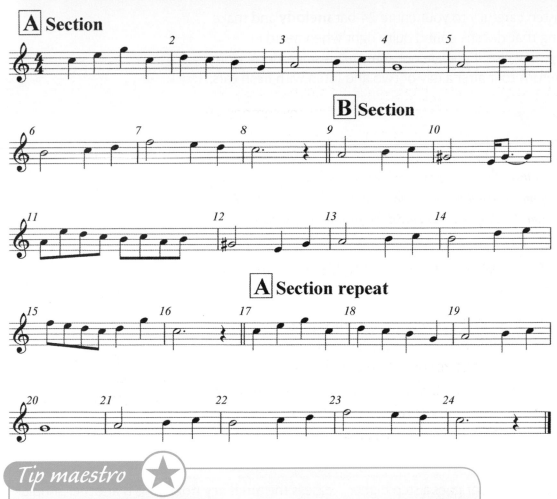

A Section

B Section

A Section repeat

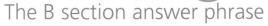

Tip maestro ⭐

Musical 'unity'

*Musical unity is achieved when all the elements of a composition (individual bars, phrases and sections) fit together convincingly as a whole — as opposed to sounding like disjointed parts that have just been stuck together. One way to create unity is to carefully re-use certain musical elements, or concepts, no matter how small — for example, a short **rhythm** fragment or a single bar. Even just a couple of notes **repeated** in various bars can maintain the logical flow of a piece.*

Activity time 26 ✏️

The B section answer phrase

Now compose a four-bar **answer** phrase for your B section, keeping in mind the concepts and techniques I have been using.

Listen to your piece

You have now completed all of the main composing – the remainder of the work will, at most, involve developing or making **variations** to what you already have.

You could of course leave your **melody** just as it is right now, in a very simple **ternary structure**. As you will see, however, it's quite easy to develop your composition into something more substantial.

You should now listen carefully to your entire 24-bar **melody** and make changes to anything that doesn't sound quite right when heard in context with everything else. If you are not sure at this stage, don't worry. Take a break and return to it after a day or two and listen with fresh ears.

> *Tip maestro*
>
> *Trust your instincts*
>
> *Don't forget the importance of trusting your instincts as you listen to your work in progress. A passage of music might be technically clever but if it doesn't fit with everything else you should either alter it or save it for another composition.*

Using musical concepts to develop your piece

In addition to the **Variation and development techniques** listed on pages 34–35, here are some other straightforward ways to extend, develop or create variety in your composition without losing musical **unity**:

- **Repeat** a bar or a passage of bars, either exactly or adding some extra notes such as *auxiliary notes, **passing notes** or **sequence** (including 'step' **sequence**).

> *An **auxiliary note** is one that goes a step higher or lower than the original note, immediately followed by the original note again. For example, F-**E**-F, C-**B**-C, G-**A**-G. The middle note in each case is the **auxiliary note**. This is another simple way to create **variation** in a **melody**, or give it more movement.

- Make occasional note changes (change the **pitch** of some of the original notes) in **repeated** bars.
- Add **first and second time bars** to repeated sections.
- Add a **coda**.
- Use musical **dynamics** including **crescendo** (**cresc.**) and **diminuendo** (**dim.**) to add expression, create **variation** at a **repeated** section, or heighten the effect of a **key change** (see also the supplementary material for this workshop at **www.jm-education.com**).

Articulation

The way individual notes are played (or articulated) can also be effective in creating **variation** as well as expressing the character of the piece.

Here are some concepts relating to the articulation of notes:
- **Legato** (smooth and sustained)
- **Staccato** (short and detached)
- **Accented** (more pronounced and slightly louder)
- **Vibrato** (where a note is 'shaken' or vibrated slightly)
- **Pitch bend** (where a note is pushed (bent) to a higher or lower pitch)

Step 7: the A section repeat, bars 17–24 (bars 1–8 repeated with variation)

The examples below show how some of the development/**variation** techniques we have looked at might be used to create new versions of the first bar of my piece. Notice how much they can alter the bar without changing its main elements. These techniques can of course be combined to create even more possibilities.

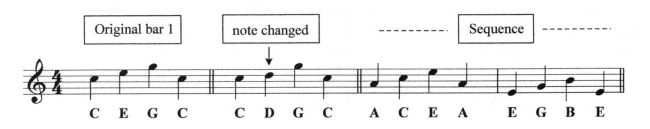

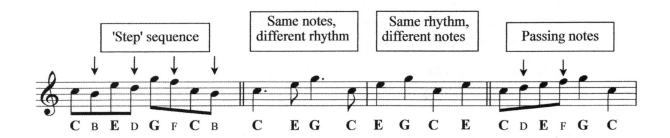

Working with these techniques I came up with two possible variations for my A section. The first is simpler, and uses mainly **rhythmic variation**. The second is more complex. Let's look at the first version.

🔊 **Listen Up: CD track 19**

Listen to the **first** version of my A section **variation** (**variation 1**) on CD track 19 as you follow the music below. When you have done this, compare **variation 1** with the original (page 36).

A Section (variation 1)

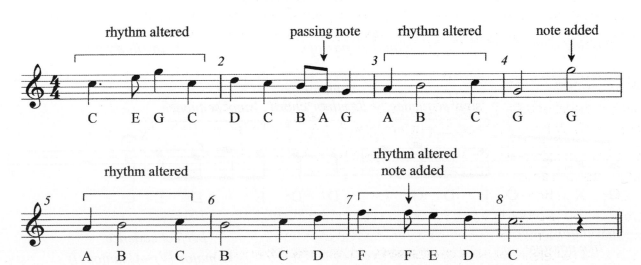

> **Concepts used to create variation: dotted rhythms, passing note.**
>
> **Summary:** Changes to the original **rhythms** are the main **variation** used, with only a single **passing note** and two extra notes added to the original melody.

For a bar-by-bar analysis see **www.jm-education.com**.

Now let's look at the second and more complex version of my A section (**variation 2**).

🔊 **Listen Up: CD track 20**

Listen to the **second** version of my A section **variation** (**variation 2**) on CD track 20 as you follow the music below. Then, compare it with the original version.

A Section (variation 2)

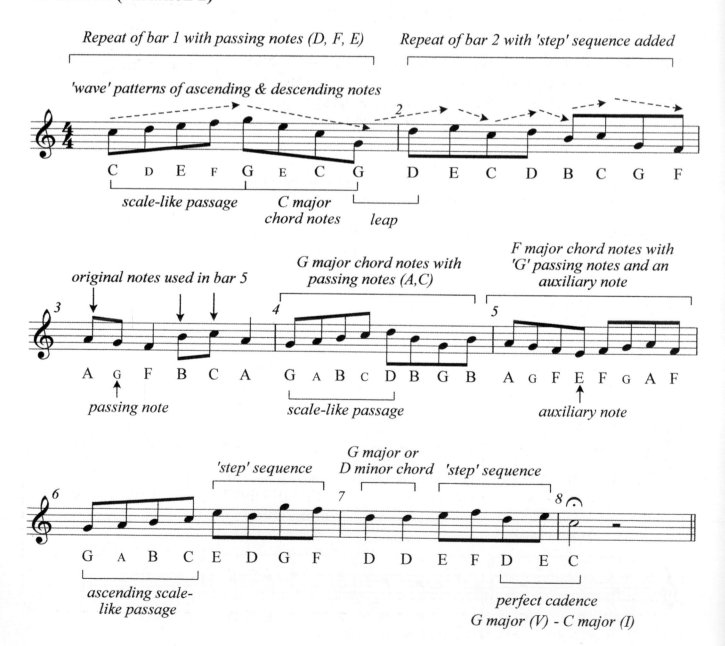

Concepts used to create variation: passing notes, 'step' sequence, chord notes.

Summary: Passing notes and 'step' sequence have been used to make this variation livelier than the original A section by producing more quaver (eighth note) note groups. Several note changes and additions have also been made.

The final four bar phrase (bars 5–8) has the most variation. Just compare these bars with those of the original A section to see what I mean. At first glance the two A sections appear to have little in common, but you will be able to hear the similarity – mainly because they are both structured from the same chords and basic melody notes.

For a bar-by-bar analysis see **www.jm-education.com**.

Almost there …

Rather than **repeat** the original version of the A section to make bars 25–32, I opted to add **variation 1** as my final section. This seemed to flow better than **variation 2**, but the whole piece was still a bit short. I tried repeating the first A and B sections to extend the composition, but this just sounded dull and unadventurous, so I tried adding A section **variation 1** again at bars 9–16, just to see how it sounded. I immediately liked it!

The B section sounded fine as it was with no **repeat**, so I left it alone. Yet the music still seemed to reach its conclusion too soon. What could I do to fix this? Would I have to compose more music to extend the last A section? Maybe. However, there was one more thing to try; it seemed too easy, but would it work if I added A section **variation 2** after **variation 1** at the end of the piece? Yes!

My final **melody**, now 40 bars long, had the following structure:

Tip maestro

Notice how **passing notes** and *auxiliary notes* can embellish and enliven your music. They are a simple and effective way to add **variation** to your composition.

A Section (C major)	B Section (A minor)	A Section repeat (C major)
Bars 1–8: A section (original) Bars 9–16: A section **(variation 1)**	Bars 17–24: B section (original)	Bars 25–32: A section **(variation 1)** Bars 33–40: A section **(variation 2)**

🔊 **Listen up: CD track 21**

Now listen to CD track 21 as you follow the music on page 44 to see what *you* think of my finished **melody**. Does the placing of my A section **variations** extend the piece effectively? Does the whole piece sound balanced? Would you have tried something different or extended the music even further?

1 The **chords** that helped me choose my **melody** notes are written above each bar. These will be very useful for the next step of the composition, **Adding accompaniment parts to the melody**. You can access this in the supplementary material for this chapter at **www.jm-education.com**.

2 The Italian term for the **tempo** – **Allegro** (**lively**) – and the precise metronome speed – ♩ = 130 (130 **crotchet** beats per minute).

You will also see that I have titled my piece simply 'Study in C'.

For a bar-by-bar analysis see **www.jm-education.com**.

Study in C

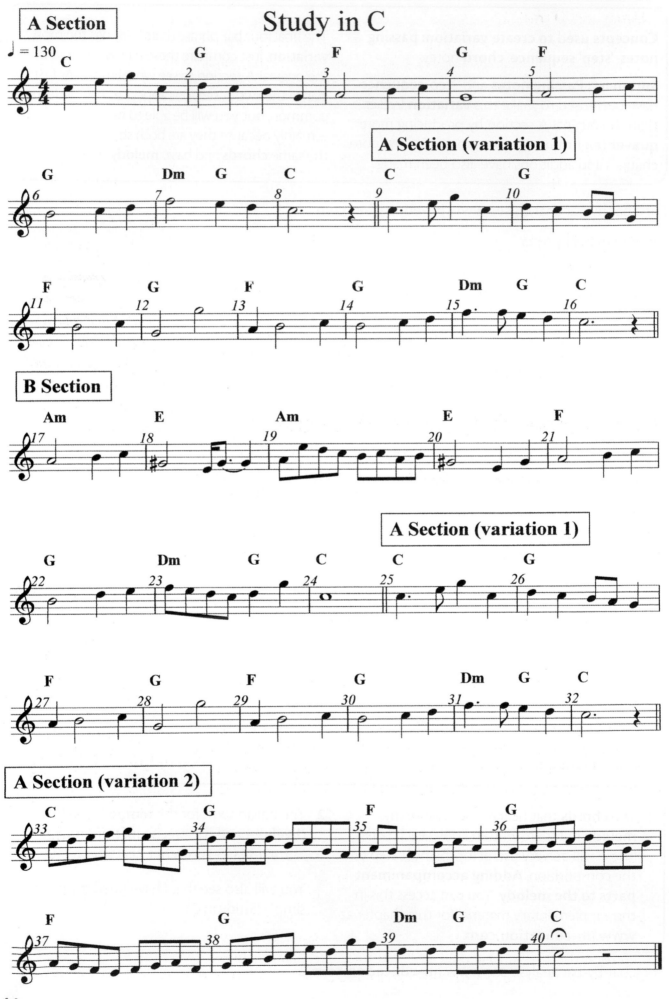

🔊 **Listen up: CD track 22**

On CD track 22 you can hear how my **melody** sounds with its three added accompaniment parts. There is a step-by-step description of how these extra parts were composed in the supplementary material for this chapter at **www.jm-education.com**.

Composing workshop 2: Composing vocal music

We are now going to explore ways to set words to music. Combined with everything you learnt in the previous workshop (composing a **melody** and **adding accompaniment parts to a melody** in the supplementary material), by the end of this workshop you should feel confident about writing an entire song complete with accompaniment. For extra guidance, you can see how a whole song was put together in the supplementary material for this vocal workshop at **www.jm-education.com**.

Which comes first, the words or the music?

As with other types of composing, there is no 'correct' way to write a song. Some songwriters never write their own words. They either have a **lyricist** who does this for them or use an existing text such as a poem. The songwriter will then write music to fit the natural **rhythm** and mood of the words. Often the songwriter and **lyricist** work together to create words and music simultaneously and the song is composed this way.

Frequently, though, a songwriter writes the words as well as the music, and the song grows from fragments of ideas – either in the form of musical notes or words – which are developed or joined together to make a complete song. This is similar to how an instrumental work might be composed, except that words are now a main part of the piece.

As with composing an instrumental piece, however, a more experienced composer or songwriter, knowing the techniques, will create a good song much quicker and more efficiently than someone who just sits around waiting for new ideas to pop into his or her head.

Here are some ways a song might be written.

- **Improvise**. Many songwriters start by sitting down with a musical instrument (usually a **keyboard** or **guitar**) and improvising with **chords** or the notes in a **scale** to generate some ideas. From this process little musical fragments or phrases are born.
- **Chords and voice**. It is quite common for songwriters to improvise with random **chords** while they sing words (either existing words or maybe improvised) until they hit upon a **chord sequence** or musical phrase they like. Other phrases will then be added that suit the style of the first.

Activity time 27 ✏️

Developing your piece

Now analyse your full **melody** and think about how it might be extended and developed. Would some **repetition**, either with or without **variation**, enhance the work further? Don't worry if nothing comes to mind straight away – your composition may be just fine as it is. Put it aside for a few days then listen to it again with fresh ears.

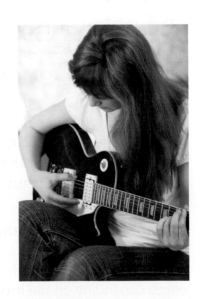

- **Music first**. Sometimes a **melody** is composed first on a musical instrument or a sequencer and the words are then written to it. **Chords** can be added at any stage, followed by other accompaniment parts such as **bass** and **drums** (if required).
- **Lyrics first**. In this case words are written (or chosen from a text) and then set to music. The main skill involved here is in creating a **melody** that reflects the mood and natural **rhythm** of the words.
- **An inspired idea**. Sometimes words or a fragment of a musical **melody** will just come into the songwriter's head, perhaps as a result of experiencing something moving or inspiring.

It is possible to build entire songs around just a single small idea if you know how. This is something the composing workshops in this book can help you with.

Tip maestro

If a great idea for a lyric (words for a song) or a melody just comes to you unexpectedly, try to get the idea down on paper or recorded quickly before it's forgotten — it is very frustrating when that inspired idea vanishes from your memory and you haven't made a note of it!

Turning words into musical phrases

For this workshop I have written a short rhyming text, which I'm going to develop into a song lyric by setting it to music.

Here is the text:

> In my darkest lonely night, you make all the stars shine bright,
> And from the sunshine in your eyes, a bright new dawn will rise.

This text might become part of a **verse** or **chorus** in a song – we don't need to know which at this stage; the important thing now is to start adding musical **rhythm** and notes to the words in order to develop a **melody**.

The natural rhythm of words

First of all, say the text out loud, as though you were actually speaking to someone in normal conversation.

When you spoke, did your voice **rise** and **fall** slightly in particular places? What kind of **rhythm** did the words create? Did you **pause** a little at each comma? And at the end did your voice **lower** to emphasise that you had finished the statement at the full stop? Say the text again and concentrate on the way your voice naturally expresses the words and shapes the overall text.

Speech, like music, has **rhythm**, **pitch**, **cadences**, **rests** (or pauses) and **dynamics** – when you are angry or excited you are likely to speak faster, louder and at a higher **pitch**, for example. Both use **phrases** that vary in length depending on the **metre** of what we are saying.

My text has its own natural **rhythm** because of the **syllables** in the words and the **punctuation** (commas and a full stop).

The **punctuation** in the text presents **two** clear structural possibilities for musical **question and answer** phrases.

Option 1

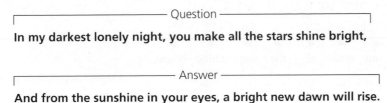

┌──────── Question ────────┐
In my darkest lonely night, you make all the stars shine bright,

┌──────── Answer ────────┐
And from the sunshine in your eyes, a bright new dawn will rise.

Or

Option 2

┌──── Question ────┐ ┌──────── Answer ────────┐
In my darkest lonely night, you make all the stars shine bright,

┌──────── Question ────────┐ ┌──── Answer ────┐
And from the sunshine in your eyes, a bright new dawn will rise.

Either option will work – and things such as note values (**rhythm**), **cadences** and the **time signature** (the number of beats in a bar) can help determine phrase structure. However, I think **option 2** best suits the natural **rhythm** of the text, so I'm going to base my **melody** on this structure.

Working out the rhythm and time signature

The first step to giving the text a basic **musical rhythm** is to place a note above each **syllable**.

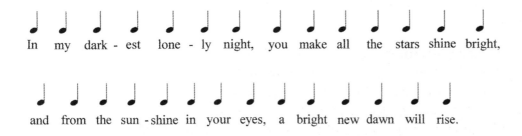

Next, we need to identify the natural **emphasis points** on the syllables. This will help us work out both **rhythm** and **time signature**. An easy way to do this is to say the phrase out loud and slowly (like a robot) to a regular beat or pulse; for example, while tapping your foot or clapping your hands in a steady, regular beat (or, better still, using a **metronome**). As you do this, listen carefully to which words are naturally more **accented**. You may need to try a few times until you feel both the beat and the words falling into place with each other. When they do, make a note of the **accented** words by placing an **accent** symbol > above them. There are two possible versions for my phrase:

Version 1

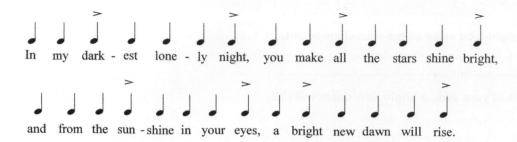

Version 2

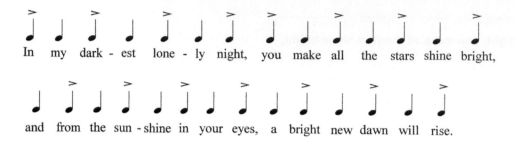

If we assume that these **accented** words represent the **first beat** of each new bar of music, we can add a bar line before them to see what kind of regular bar pattern emerges.

Version 1

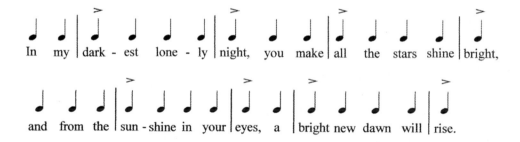

In **version 1** the **accents** mostly fall every **four** syllables, so we could have four bars of music, each with four main beats, giving us a **4/4 time signature**. In those bars that have less than four notes we can use longer note values or **rests** to maintain the regular four-beat pattern.

Version 2

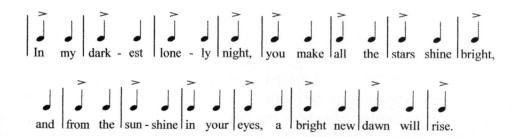

In **version 2** the **accents** mostly fall every **two** syllables, in which case we could have eight bars of music, each with two main beats, giving us a **2/4 time signature**. Again, in any bars that have just one note we can use longer note values or **rests** to maintain the regular two-beat pattern.

I think a **2/4 time signature** seems less likely as the words don't really fit with a two-beat 'feel' – which is often used for **marches**. So I'm going with a **4/4 time signature**.

Other **time signatures** are possible, but there is no benefit in making things more complex than necessary at present. Besides, some of the best songs ever written are in **4/4 time** – it's not called 'common time' for nothing!

Anacrusis

You will notice that the version I am going to use (**version 1**) does not begin with an accented syllable – it does not start on the first beat of the bar. This means the musical phrase will start with an **anacrusis**.

Developing the rhythm

Now that the basic phrase structure has been worked out I can set about creating a more interesting and expressive **rhythm** for the words (at present every syllable is represented only by a **crotchet** or quarter note). This might require some experimentation until we find the **rhythm** we like but, as a guide, it is common in songs to have a **longer note value** or a **rest** where there is a natural pause in the words – for example at a **comma** or **full stop**, or at the end of a **question** or **answer** phrase. (Don't forget that pauses in the music also allow the singer to take a breath.)

So we could have a **rhythm** something like this:

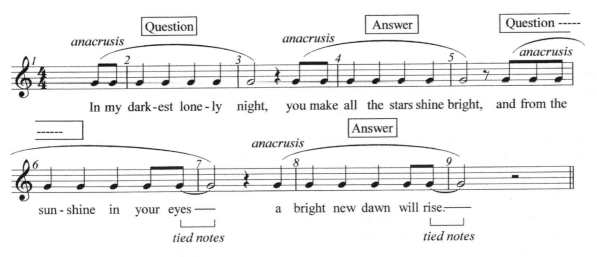

1 For clarity the **rhythm** has been shown on a musical stave using a repeating note, **G**, with lyrics underneath. I will work on the **pitches** in the next section, **Choosing the notes**.

2 The curved lines above the music are **phrase lines** indicating the beginning and end of

each musical phrase (the **question and answer** phrases I mapped out earlier).

3 The musical phrase structure and my **rhythm** choices have resulted in four examples of **anacrusis**.

I have added longer note values (**minims** or **half notes**) at the end of each **question and answer** phrase followed by a **rest** to emphasise the natural pauses, while the shorter note values (**quavers** or **eighth notes**) in bars 1, 3, 5, 6 and 8 further break up the repetitiveness of the steady **crotchet** (**quarter note**) beats. Notice also the **tied notes** in bars 6–7 and 8–9; this is a simple technique (also used in workshop 1, pages 37 and 39), that can make a **rhythm** much more interesting.

🔊 Listen up: CD track 23

Listen to this **rhythm** now on CD track 23 as you follow the notation above. A metronome click emphasises the first beats in the bar.

These simple adjustments to the **rhythm** have already given the phrase real musical shape, and we don't need to stop there. In songs we have much more freedom to play around with words than we do when speaking. For example, a single word or syllable might last for several seconds (if it has a long or **tied note** value), or a fraction of that (**staccato**), and it could be sung to one note (**syllabic**) or several in succession (**melismatic**).

It can be enjoyable experimenting with the possibilities. Below are two other possible **rhythms** for my musical phrase.

In this second version I have introduced **dotted rhythms** (**dotted crotchet** or **dotted quarter notes**) and added more **quavers** (**eighth notes**).

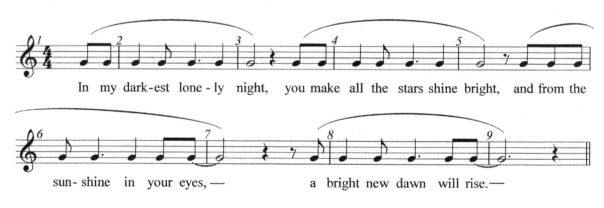

🔊 Listen up: CD track 24

Listen to this new version on CD track 24 now as you follow the notation above. Compare it to the original on CD track 23.

The next version is a bit more complex, and makes more use of **syncopation**.

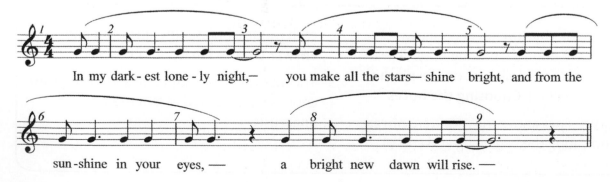

◄))) Listen up: CD track 25

Listen to this **rhythm** on CD track 25 now as you follow the notation above, then compare it with the two previous **rhythms** on CD tracks 23 and 24. Can you hear the **syncopation** in this latest version?

Activity time 28 🖉

Practice makes perfect

Using existing lines of text (such as poetry) or words you have made up yourself, repeat the previous steps of adding musical **rhythm** to various short phrases.

With practice, you should begin to feel confident about writing a complete song.

Of course, organising my words into structured musical phrases complete with a **time signature** and some **rhythm** options *first*, even before I have thought about note **pitches**, is not the only way I could have begun. Another alternative would have been to work out the **rhythm** and notes simultaneously on a musical instrument, recording or writing down each step. However, as in workshop 1, my aim is to show you some solid techniques that will produce structured pieces of music while avoiding any unnecessary difficulties. These techniques are useful to know if you are new to composing or get stuck at any point in the process. But they can be effective for experienced composers too — consider that all I have to do now is alter the note pitches in my phrase and I will have a flawless line of music for a new song.

And of course there are techniques for doing that, too ...

Choosing the notes

Two important considerations when setting words to music are the **key** and **pitch**.

Key

Whether **major** or **minor**, the key needs to reflect the mood of the words. Serious or sad lyrics would be best expressed in a **minor key**, whereas a **major key** will suit happy, light-hearted words. We can of course **change key** during the course of the song, perhaps by setting the **chorus** in a different key to the **verses**.

A **major key** suits the mood of my words, so I chose **G major**. The **scale** notes in this key can be found on page 20, **Scales and key signatures**. For more detailed information (including basic chords in this key) see the companion website at **www.jm-education.com**.

Pitch

The **pitch** of the notes is important for two reasons. First, a rise or fall (or a **leap**) in **pitch** helps to shape a musical phrase and express emotion just as it does in speech. Second, we have to be careful that the notes can be sung comfortably and are therefore not too high or too low for the intended voice range. This range will of course depend on the singer (male or female, child or adult, amateur or professional), but you should at least be able to sing your own song! If in doubt, try singing the intended notes and phrases of a song yourself before declaring it finished.

As a general 'safe' range, choose notes that are *on* or very close to being on the musical stave, avoiding those with **leger lines**. (See **Notes on the treble clef stave**, page 18, for this 'safe' range of notes.)

Now that I have the **key** selected and an awareness of the vocal range, I can start choosing my notes.

Cadences

You may remember in workshop 1 that we began with the notes of the **cadences** first as these provided both structure and a reference point for the other notes.

Thanks to the **question and answer** phrase structure my **cadence** points are easy to spot. (They often are in vocal music.) I decided to have an **imperfect cadence** at the end of both **question** phrases and a **perfect cadence** at the end of the **answer** phrases.

To achieve this, at the **cadence** points in my **melody** I just had to choose notes from the **cadence chord** I want to use. For example, if I want a **I–V imperfect cadence**, my note choices for **chord I** (**G major**) are G, B and D, and for **chord V** (**D major**) they are D, F# and A. (For more on **cadences** refer to workshop 1 and the companion website **www.jm-education.com**.)

Alternatively, you might use the simpler 'rule of thumb' approach to creating **cadences**, which is: end a phrase on the **key note** to make a **perfect cadence**, end it on any note *except* a key note to make a simplistic version of an **imperfect cadence**. Remember, though, that a proper imperfect cadence should end on a note used in **chord V**. Accompaniment **chords** that harmonise with the **melody** notes can then be added later.

Activity time 29

Another way to choose the notes …

To work out suitable melodies for their lyrics, songwriters often sing the words to improvised tunes until they find something suitable.

Try singing my song lyrics to some of your own improvised tunes. Start by making up your own **rhythm**, but then try singing or improvising in the **rhythm** of one (or all three) of my **rhythm** options above (use the CD tracks to help you – or try singing in **unison** with these recorded **rhythms**). As you improvise, experiment with changing the **pitch** of your voice (**ascending** and **descending**) to suit the phrase lengths and **cadence** points.

This method often results in 'ready-made' phrases whose note names you can work out on a musical instrument and then set down in standard notation.

Here are my three **rhythm** versions with notes added to each. My
chord choices appear above the **melodies**; notice how these create the
imperfect and **perfect cadences**.

Listen up: CD track 26

Follow the **melody** of the completed song phrase below as you listen to
it on CD track 26. This **melody** was developed from the **rhythm** heard
on CD track 23.

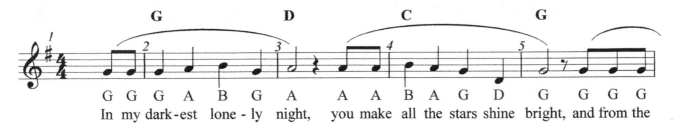
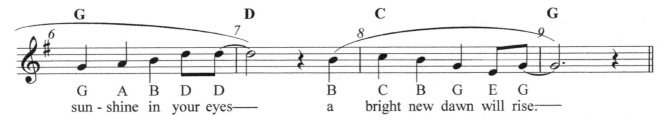

Listen up: CD track 27

Follow the **melody** of the completed song phrase below as you listen to
it on CD track 27. This **melody** was developed from the **rhythm** heard
on CD track 24. (There are two small alterations: I added a **melisma** in bar
7 and an **A minor chord** in bar 8.)

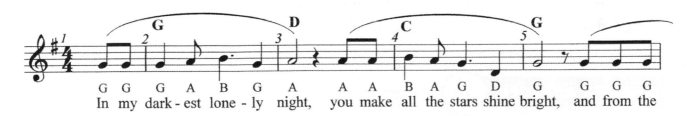
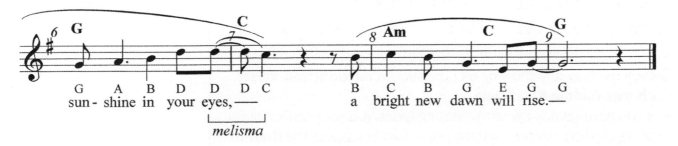

Listen up: CD track 28

Follow the **melody** of the completed song phrase below as you listen to
it on CD track 28. This **melody** was developed from the **rhythm** heard
on CD track 25. (I use a **melisma** in bar 7 here too, as well as an **A minor
chord** in bar 8.)

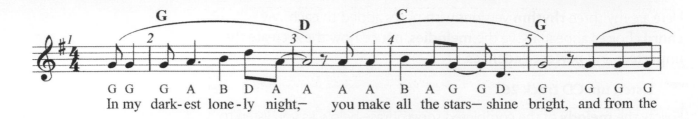

G G G A B D A A A A B A G G D G G G G
In my dark-est lone-ly night,— you make all the stars— shine bright, and from the

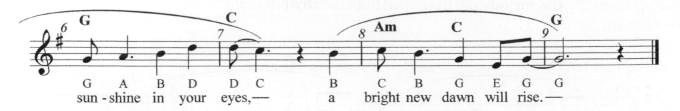

G A B D D C B C B G E G G
sun-shine in your eyes,— a bright new dawn will rise.—

I can now use one of these completed phrases as a solid starting point from which to develop a full song.

Activity time 30

Finish my song

Choose one of the finished phrases above and, based on the techniques we have looked at in this chapter, compose others to go with it, gradually transforming it into a full song. Feel free to change any aspect of the original **melody** or **lyrics** if you wish.

Before tackling this exercise, you will find it helpful to complete the supplementary workshop **Analysing a modern song** on the companion website **www.jm-education.com**. In this workshop you will look at the various component parts of a full modern song, complete with **lyrics**, analysing and listening to each step of its composition.

If you want to get started on your song straight away, however, the remainder of this chapter has some helpful pieces of information, reminders, tips and exercises to help you on your way.

Concepts at work

Song composing: quick reference points and suggestions 1

★ You might map out a basic structure plan for your entire song to begin with, clearly showing sections such as **introduction**, **verses**, **chorus**, **middle 8** and **coda**.

★ If you have already chosen your song **lyrics**, you may find it helpful to divide this text into metered phrases and compose the **rhythm** first, just as we did in this workshop.

★ Before choosing musical notes for your **lyrics**, try singing them first with **improvised** notes in a **rhythm** you have already composed, just to see whether any melodic ideas pop into your head.

⇨

* A song's **chorus** is usually more memorable or 'catchy' than its **verses**. It might, for example, **change key**.
* A **coda** can be a convenient way to take you out of a **verse** or **chorus** and end your song smoothly.
* **Instrumental** sections and **middle 8** (**bridge**) passages not only provide a link between sections (for example, joining a **verse** with the **chorus**), but also add interest and variety to a song.

Song composing: quick reference points and suggestions 2

* Choose a musical **key** or **keys** that reflect the mood or the changing mood of the song.
* Think about adding the **cadence** notes first to ensure a logical structure.
* Consider how your lyrical phrases might naturally **ascend** or **descend** in **pitch**.
* A common song structure alternates between **verses** and a repeating **chorus**.
* Each **verse** and **chorus** is on average about **four phrases** long, although this is variable.
* Each **verse** normally has different lyrics but those of the **chorus** stay the same.

Tip maestro

*Well-chosen musical **dynamics** – including **crescendos** and **diminuendos** – add expression to (and therefore enhance the meaning of) a song's lyrics, just as a good speaker can make a story come alive in the way they speak the words.*

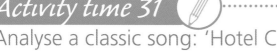

Activity time 31

Analyse a classic song: 'Hotel California' by The Eagles

As you will understand by now, one of the best ways to learn about music is to *listen* to it and hear all those concepts and techniques being used by experienced, professional musicians.

For this exercise I'd like you to listen to a famous song, 'Hotel California' by The Eagles, and analyse its structure. I have chosen this song because it has good examples of some characteristic elements commonly used in popular songs. These are listed below. Listen out for them carefully then, after hearing the song a few more times, see if you can add any more concepts to the list.

* **Instrumental introduction** or '**intro**'.
* **Verses** and **chorus** have a clear **question and answer** structure.
* The **chorus** is livelier than the **verses**.
* The **chorus** is in a different **key** (**major**) to the **verses** (**minor**), making it more 'catchy' and memorable.
* There is an **instrumental section** played by lead **guitar** (quite a long one in this case).

Tip maestro

As with all kinds of music study, listening plays a huge part. If you want to write a song, listen to lots of songs and note the structure of the phrases, and how key, musical notes and dynamics express the lyrics. Then, go and write your own great song!

Activity time 32

Analyse some of your favourite songs

Now that you've had some analysis practice with 'Hotel California' in the Activity time above, it's time to try the same thing on some of your favourite songs. As you listen to each song of your choice, make a note of its main features.

Things to listen for are:

- Is there an **introduction**?
- Can you tell how many vocal phrases there are in each **verse**?
- Do the phrases have a **question and answer** structure?
- Are there **ascending** and **descending** passages in the **melody**?
- Do the **verses** have a regular length or are some longer or shorter than others?
- Is the song in a **major key** or a **minor key**? Does it **change key** at any point?
- Is the **chorus** livelier than the **verses**? Does it change **key**?
- Is there a **middle 8** section?
- Is there an **instrumental** section?
- Does the song have a **coda**?

You will probably hear some other features/concepts too – and don't be surprised if you notice things that you were unaware of before doing this exercise.

Tip maestro

An *introduction* or 'intro' is the opening section of a song (usually instrumental), normally between four and eight bars long and often consisting of a **chord sequence** that is used in the song itself. For this reason *intros* are often easier to write when your song is finished as you will already have all the **chord sequences** worked out. An example of an *intro* occurs in the song that is analysed in the supplementary composing workshop at *www. jm-education.com*.

Concepts at work

Key changes in songs

Many songs have a **key change** in them – perhaps halfway through, or at the **chorus**, for example. A **key change** can create contrast, add greater emphasis to the lyrics or alter the mood. Changing from a **major key** to a **minor key** might inject a solemn mood into a song that has begun pleasantly, whereas changing to a **major key** after beginning in a **minor key** will work perfectly if, for instance, you are singing about someone whose life was boring until they met the person of their dreams! Listen to some songs about relationships – those that are good and those that have gone bad – and notice how the songwriters use musical **keys** to express the mood of the lyrics.

Here are a few examples to get you started. Find these songs online and listen carefully for the **key changes**.

- ★ 'You Raise Me Up' by **Westlife** (cover version)
- ★ 'Blaze of Glory' by **Bon Jovi**
- ★ 'Every Breath You Take' by **Sting**

Activity time 33

Once you have completed your composition, make sure you get it recorded, either using a **sequencer** or live musicians. Remember, you owe it to yourself to have a permanent record of all the work you put into transforming a simple **melody** into a unique, fully harmonised and original piece of music.

Tip maestro

*One of the best (and easiest) things you can do to help yourself with composing and improvising is to **listen** to lots of different kinds of music. Even a style you don't especially enjoy could give you some ideas that you might be able to use in your creative musical work.*

Composing review

Don't forget – of the 30 marks (15% of the overall course award) available for the composing assignment, 10 of those (5% of the overall course award) are awarded for the review component.

The SQA state that, in the composing review, candidates must:

- provide a detailed account of the main decisions when exploring and developing their musical ideas
- identify strengths and/or areas which could be improved

The composing review can be presented in prose or bullet points and as a guide should be in the region of 200 to 300 words. However, word count is only given to indicate the volume of evidence required. No penalty will be applied.

Although this is something that your teacher will be best placed to advise and guide you on, it is worth providing a brief example review here, just to give you an idea of the sorts of things you might want to include.

Stimulus
I wanted to compose a piece of instrumental music that incorporates some of the musical concepts I have been studying in National 5 Music. The instrumental dances of the Baroque period interested me, so I decided to write a lively work in Rondo form with a ground bass.
Resources
Piano, violin, manuscript paper and MIDI keyboard linked to a computer running a DAW (Digital Audio Workstation)
Significant decisions
I wanted to write a Rondo that could be performed either as a trio or as a piano and violin duet (mainly because these are two instruments I play myself). The ground bass and chord parts of my Rondo can be played on two separate instruments or piano (one part for each hand), while the melody is suited to an instrument (such as violin) capable of sustaining notes in a lyrical way.
Process
I began by making a list of all the things I wanted to include in this piece (ground bass, keys, chords, passing notes, etc.), as well as writing a structure plan. I composed a basic two-bar ground bass figure first, which is repeated with occasional variation throughout the Rondo. I then wrote the first four-bar phrase of the melody by experimenting/improvising with the scale of C major. I went on to create the other main sections of my Rondo by experimenting with the scales of G major and A minor, as well as re-using some of the material from the first four-bar phrase. Last of all, I composed the middle part, the chord accompaniment, using the melody and ground bass as a guide to chord choice.
Strengths/areas which could be improved
I would say the strength of this piece is that it has a solid structure that makes it flow from start to finish. It also uses musical concepts in a carefully-considered, structured way. If there is an area that could be improved it is perhaps the middle chord part, which is a bit simple. Here, I could have experimented more with different chords and rhythms.

Chapter 5

Performing

Musical performance is one of the most important parts of the National 5 Music course. It carries **50%** of the total marks available. This practical activity offers students the opportunity to gain experience in two musical instruments (or one instrument plus voice) selected from a large list (see below), and will be overseen largely by a course teacher and/or instrumental tutor. This chapter therefore focuses on related aspects such as the course requirements and what examiners will be assessing you on, as well as advice on things like effective practising, performing strategies, tackling the final exam and coping with performance nerves.

You will normally choose your performance programme assisted by a class teacher or music tutor who can advise you on appropriate music, but a guide to the standard required and a list of suggested pieces for each instrument (at grade 3 level) can be found at the following source:

- SQA's **National Qualifications in Music: Performing** at **www.sqa.org.uk**.

Grade 3 level practical exam syllabuses are available online at the following centres:
- The Associated Board of the Royal Schools of Music (ABRSM) **www.abrsm.org**.
- Trinity College **www.trinitycollege.co.uk**.
- London College of Music **www.uwl.ac.uk/academic-schools/music**.
- The Royal Conservatoire of Scotland (RCS) Scottish Traditional Music Grade Exams **www.rcs.ac.uk**.

Course requirements

During your National 5 Music course you will have the opportunity to perform on **two** different musical instruments or a musical instrument and voice. This could involve **solo** playing and/or playing as part of a group of musicians.

Your options are to perform **solo** and/or **as part of a group** in one of these combinations:
- **two** musical instruments
- **one** musical instrument **and** voice
- **one** solo musical instrument **and** a different instrument **as part of a group**
- **solo voice** and an instrument **as part of a group**

You can choose from **two** of the following instruments (including voice):

Accordion (Free bass or Stradella)	Organ (Pipe)
Bagpipes (Scottish)	Piano
Baritone and Euphonium	Pipe Band Drumming
Bassoon	Recorder (Descant)
Bass guitar	Recorder (Treble)
Cello	Saxophone (Alto and Baritone)
Clarinet	Saxophone (Soprano and Tenor)
Clàrsach	Scots Fiddle
Cornet (E flat)	Snare Drum
Double bass	Timpani
Drum kit	Tin Whistle
Flute	Trombone (Tenor)
Guitar (Classical)	Trumpet (B flat Cornet and Flugel)
Guitar (Acoustic and Electric)	Tuba
Harp	Tuned Percussion
Horn in F	Ukelele
Horn (Tenor)	Viola
Keyboard (Electronic)	Violin
Oboe	Voice

Some instrument combinations are not permitted. For example, two instruments from the same family, such as two keyboard instruments or bass guitar and double bass. For clarification refer to **Music: Performing – Grid of Approved Combinations of Instruments** on the SQA website: **www.sqa.org.uk**.

Assessment

Towards the end of your course you will prepare a programme of music lasting between **8** and **8½** minutes that is played live to an examiner. Your performance can be in a **solo** or a **group** setting, or both, and makes up 50% of the total marks available.

The performance time on either instrument must be at least **2** minutes and you should perform at least **two** contrasting pieces on each instrument.

You will be assessed on:
- your ability to perform a programme of solo music and/or respond to others in a group
- your ability to maintain musical flow and realise the composer's intentions
- melodic accuracy/intonation
- rhythmic accuracy
- maintaining the **tempo** of the music
- demonstrating musicality through mood and character and tone
- **dynamics**

Get some performing help

A music tutor

An ideal way to learn to play a musical instrument is to get lessons from an experienced teacher. You might think you can teach yourself but you will not have the experience to identify or tackle a problem effectively when it arises, nor can you watch yourself from a distance as you play with the practised eye of a good teacher. This is why a lot of people who start teaching themselves give up after a while as they don't see themselves improving, or find some techniques too difficult to master. It's not because they have no ability for the instrument, or were necessarily attempting practical things that were too difficult, but because they did not have a teacher who could advise them on how to overcome the problem. For example, difficulty with stretching to a note on a stringed instrument often has more to do with the way a person is sitting or holding the instrument than the length of their fingers. An experienced teacher can identify the cause of such problems and will have solutions to overcome them.

However, it may be that you are not able to get lessons from a tutor, or just want to try an instrument to see if you like it, in which case you have the following options.

The internet

A wealth of music learning resources exist online, including recorded lessons from tutors, playing advice, and easy chord and *tab arrangements of thousands of songs and pieces of music. Personal tuition and advice is available at **www.yourmusicmentor.com**. (*Tab, an abbreviation of **tablature**, is a means of writing a piece of music using a number system to show where the notes are on a musical instrument without the requirement to read music.)

If, for example, you want to learn to play the keyboard you can see just how much help is available by typing 'keyboard online lessons' into an internet search bar.

Tutor books

A lot of tutor books are aimed at beginners looking to try out a musical instrument for themselves. Many come with instructional DVDs and internet links for an interactive experience that could be the next best thing to having a private tutor. Don't be tempted to rush through the pages in an attempt to progress quickly, though: work carefully and methodically to make sure you have really grasped each new thing you need to learn so that none of the steps become too difficult.

If you do opt for tutor books and/or internet resources, remember that any problems you encounter in mastering a technique or a chord shape may have nothing to do with the fact that you have no aptitude for a particular instrument – it could be that you just need a little expert advice.

The importance of practice

We've all been told that 'practice makes perfect', but it really is the most important part of learning to play a musical instrument. It is the one thing that a teacher, the internet or a book cannot do for you, yet it requires about 80% of your total time commitment in the learning process (the other 20% is actual tuition). To put it another way, if an average lesson lasts half an hour you should allocate half an hour to practise each day if you want to progress well.

There is no substitute for regular practice. You can't 'cram' your daily routine into a single long session since it is the regular, everyday working of muscles (or breathing) and **repetition** of playing that makes you improve. You might know how the piece should sound, and what the notes, **chords** and **rhythms** are, but without having physically worked through it several times, you will not be able to play it fluently – unless it's really simple and you happen to be an amazing sight reader! (Long practice sessions after a period of inactivity can even injure your voice or hand muscles, just as you could expect to pull a muscle if you ran a sprint without warming up first.)

Sticking to a daily practice routine requires some self-discipline, but you will be well rewarded for your efforts when you see and hear yourself steadily improving. And the better you can play an instrument, the more pleasure you will get from the experience.

So, if you are the kind of person who tends to leave studying or revision to the last minute, it's time to change your approach – you won't be able to do this in music performance.

Tip maestro

*Practice helps make playing 'automatic'. This increases your technical **skill** and **fluency** and therefore your **confidence** when performing live.*

Some key points to remember

- Try to practise every day. You will progress more quickly and play well more consistently – in other words, make fewer mistakes! Practising for half an hour every day is much better than an hour every second day, or 2 hours each day at the weekend. As in sport, this type of practice routine is the key to performing well consistently.
- Even on days when you really don't have much time, at least try to do **something**. Taking a few minutes to play one piece of music is better than no practice at all.
- You should not begin a practice session with technically demanding work as you will play better after having warmed up first. It is frustrating when, for example, your fingers don't move as efficiently as you want them to because they are 'cold' – which won't do your confidence any good either. So start easy and build up.
- Weaknesses in your playing are magnified when you feel under pressure – for example, when playing in front of people, or in an exam. That's why it's so important to spend some time focusing on the more

difficult parts of your music when practising. Your goal is to make these tricky bits the easiest – for this reason it often helps if you can commit them to memory.

Making practice enjoyable

There are times when practice can be a bit of a chore, even for experienced professional musicians. However, more often than not it is the **thought** of having to practise, not the actual practising itself, that puts us off.

When approached in the correct way, practising music isn't homework, it's an escape into a creative world where you can express yourself in your own unique way while constantly improving your skills.

Every time you practise can be an enjoyable and rewarding experience if you know some ways to keep these sessions fresh. Practising should be a routine but the *way* you practise need not be. Try some of these tactics to stay motivated:

- Ease yourself into practice. Begin with exercises such as **scales** or light **improvisation** to get yourself focused and your muscles (or voice) warmed up before concentrating on more challenging music.
- Vary the order in which you do things in a practice session. You can, for example, separate a piece of music into sections and work on these in **any order** before eventually joining up the whole thing properly. Learning the last line of a piece of music **first** might seem a bit mad, but the novelty will hold your attention – and you will still be doing the job of learning the piece.
- Always allocate some of your practice time to playing music you have already mastered (a piece from your repertoire) and to just having a bit of fun – perhaps by playing/singing along to some of your favourite songs or improvising to a backing track (these come with some music books and are also available on the internet).
- Music can be a very social activity, so why not get together with other musicians now and then to share your music and practise techniques – maybe even form a band?

Getting ready to perform in the exam

Playing to an audience, even if it's just one person, can be a daunting if not totally nerve-wracking prospect. Being well prepared is a sure way to build confidence in your own ability and keep those nerves under control – again, this is all down to your daily practice. However, there are some other things you can do to help make it less scary.

Tip maestro

Remember, there is no short cut to learning to play a musical instrument well apart from practising. You can't buy a practice app or hire someone to do it for you! However, that doesn't mean it has to feel like homework. You can still practise properly and enjoy yourself.

Tip maestro

The ability to play an instrument, or sing well, is not a skill that everyone has. People admire musical talent. Performing music is therefore something that will earn you the admiration of others and a sense of pride in yourself. So, next time you grumble about having to practise, just remember what you are getting in return!

Two good ways to prepare for live performances

1 Put yourself under some pressure …

Play in front of other people as often as you can. Ask friends or family (or anyone who is willing) to listen to a piece you have learned and can play well. Begin with music that shows you in the best light then later, as your confidence grows, play something you are still working on – or just a section of it – and afterwards listen to the feedback of your audience. The important point of this exercise is not to collect compliments but to get some experience playing for someone other than yourself.

Take on board any constructive comments your listeners may have, but don't feel dejected if they criticise – they may just be trying to help you with what little knowledge they have of what you are doing.

You don't even have to get people to sit down and watch as you play; just playing within their earshot will still put you in the situation of playing before a 'live audience' – while taking the pressure off yourself a little by the fact that they are not staring at you.

However you go about it, playing in front of others will help you grow accustomed to performing with people just *being* there. Give it time and you will learn to focus even when you have that nervy feeling in your stomach.

2 Record yourself

Make an audio recording of your exam pieces or, better still, film yourself playing them if you can. Doing this has two benefits: first, it will put you under a bit of pressure and therefore in a similar situation to being in an exam room; and second, you will be able to analyse your own playing when you listen to/watch the recording. Did it sound or look like you knew what you were doing? Was it a confident performance? Were your posture and technique good?

You can then work on improving any areas that seemed weak until you get a performance you are happy with. When you are, you could perhaps upload the excerpt to a social website for your friends to hear/see and comment on. Setting yourself a goal like this might be the ideal motivation to improve your technique and overall performance presentation. It will also help you combat any confidence or embarrassment issues you feel about solo performing. It can be tough at first, but sticking with it will help.

One word of advice, though: when you record yourself, wait for a day or so before listening to/watching the recording. You are likely to be overly critical of your playing if you listen to it immediately. If you wait a while you will be able to analyse it more objectively (and fairly).

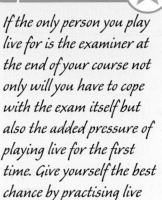

Tip maestro

If the only person you play live for is the examiner at the end of your course not only will you have to cope with the exam itself but also the added pressure of playing live for the first time. Give yourself the best chance by practising live performance.

One week before the exam

To avoid any unnecessary pressure in the days leading up to your exam:

- Make sure that your programme of music is prepared and ready to be performed *at least* a week before the exam. By this stage you should only be keeping your pieces 'warm' by playing them every day; there should be nothing left to learn or improve on.
- Find out the time and place of your exam so there is no confusion on the day. Also, ensure you will have a place where you can warm up before going into the exam room.
- Make any necessary preparations for the exam, such as copying music, ensuring your instrument is in good condition (if necessary, replace old strings on a stringed instrument with fresh ones at least a week before the exam) and, if you will be using an accompanist, make him or her aware of the place and time of the exam and arrange a few practice sessions together. Practising regularly with a backing track (if applicable) is also useful.
- Make sure you get plenty of rest the night before the exam. Lack of sleep increases stress on your body and affects your concentration.

The morning of the exam

- Don't underestimate the importance of good food. It is fuel for concentration, alertness, energy levels and even mood. Remember that caffeine in tea, coffee and energy drinks can sometimes make people feel on edge or even shake – which will aggravate any symptoms of nervousness. Drinking water will prevent a dry mouth when you're nervous, and this will be especially important if you are going to be singing.
- Get to the exam room in plenty of time. Being in the area of the exam room well before your scheduled time will avoid the danger of becoming stressed from running late.
- Have a warm up before the exam, but not more than about half an hour. Any longer might take the edge off your exam performance.

Tip maestro

Examiners are scary people: true or false?

Some facts you should know about these mysterious people known as 'Music Examiners' ...

False: Music Examiners like nothing more than to see students squirm and tremble as they play through their programme of music.

True: Music Examiners are experienced musicians who are highly sympathetic to how nervous you might feel since they have been in the same situation many times themselves. (You have to take a lot of exams to become an examiner!)

False: Because they are employed by an examination board, Music Examiners are big-headed judges who make sure that all mistakes in a performance are punished by the deduction of marks.

$\Rightarrow$

True: The policy of the Music Examiner, and the music examination board, is to reward students with marks for every good aspect of their performance rather than deduct them for every mistake they make.

False: Music Examiners were teased at school by jealous classmates who could hardly play a note and this has made them vengeful of all students who give performances that are not perfect.

True: Music Examiners *want* to give you marks. They *want* you to pass.

False: An examiner once said to a student, 'I hate teenagers'.

True: An examiner once said to a student, 'Don't worry about making the odd mistake. It's all the good stuff I will be listening out for.'

False: If you make a mistake and carry on like nothing has happened the examiner will think, 'nice try, but you can't hide anything from me ...'.

True: Dealing well with a mistake by carrying on unfazed will impress the examiner as this shows a professional attitude.

False: Music Examiners have such high standards that they find performance errors annoying.

True: Music Examiners are accustomed to hearing all kinds of mistakes and performing slips. They expect them because they know the pressure of the exam situation can cause them. However, they can also usually tell which mistakes are caused by performance nerves and which are the result of insufficient practice. So be warned!

The performance exam

- Don't be in a rush to start playing; take some time to make sure things are set up the way you want. Is the music stand at the correct height? Can you see the music clearly? If you are using a chair, is it positioned well in front of the music stand? If you are playing piano, is the stool at the best height for you? You put a lot of work into preparing for this day so give yourself every advantage to play at your best.

- Don't ponder the possibility of making mistakes; commit yourself to showing the examiner what you can do and **go for it**!

- Just before you begin playing each piece, think about the opening few seconds of the music. This can prevent 'false starts' when you have to stop and begin again.

- Your music only comes alive if you play with feeling, so get into the mood and character of each piece as you play. Playing with genuine feeling transmits to the listener; if you feel it they will too. A performance that has some mistakes but is played with feeling is likely to get more marks than one that is technically flawless but emotionless.

Tip maestro

*Dynamics are like a storyteller's voice. Loud (**f**) can express anger, power, drama; quiet (**p**) can be calm, gentle, relaxing. Having the contrast of both gives character to a piece of music.*

Group performing

All of the material in this chapter is also relevant to group performing. However, there are a few other things to consider when working with a group of musicians.

- Try to be a team player. Everyone in a music group contributes to the overall sound, which means no performer is more important than another. If every member wants to be the coolest, or the front man, it can destroy the band. Bad attitudes often make for bad music, so keep the egos at bay!
- Regular rehearsals make for rapid progress and a better standard of music. Everyone should treat rehearsals with respect, turning up on time every time. The reward will be enjoyable music and a group to be proud of.
- Make sure you can be heard clearly during the exam – you may be playing in a group, but the examiner/assessor must be able to hear your playing. Do a careful sound check before the performance.

Some extra advice on performing live

Performance nerves

When he was asked how he overcomes performance nerves one world-class musician commented, 'I haven't overcome them and I never will. I just practise until I can play my music at 120% so that when the nerves shave off a chunk in live play I'm still averaging about 100%.'

This comment shows that even top professionals experience nerves. Knowing how to cope with them is part of being a successful performer.

So here are a few helpful bits of information:

- It is perfectly normal to be a little nervous before a performance. It is even desirable – it will help keep your mind focused on the task ahead.
- Begin your performance with a piece you find a bit easier to play than the others. This will allow for any 'jitters' at the start that might affect a more challenging piece. *Never* be tempted to play your most technically demanding music at the start just to 'get it out of the way.'
- Don't expect to 'cure' yourself of performance nerves. You won't. The best any performer can do is get used to the feeling so that it doesn't become overwhelming.
- Few people play as well in front of an audience as they do when they are on their own and the pressure is off. Accept this fact and never beat yourself up with comments like, 'I can play that song perfectly – why did I make so many mistakes today?'

Tip maestro

Every bad experience presents an opportunity for a better one

Occasionally, performers have a bad day when things just don't go right or nerves affect their performance. If this happens to you don't worry about it. It can happen to even the best, most famous artists at times. Consider the experience a valuable lesson that will allow you to analyse what went wrong and take steps to reduce the chances of it happening again. Use weak performances to motivate you to do better next time rather than make you feel bad about yourself.

It is more important for you to gain performing experience (of all kinds) than to play flawlessly every time. The only way to get that experience is to keep on playing. A bad performance doesn't make a bad musician.

Playing in front of lots of people looking at us, playing to an examiner who is assessing us, being scared that we won't play our best because we feel nervous, making embarrassing mistakes, worrying that our feelings of insecurity will show on our face – all these things concern most players at some stage.

Now that you know how to prepare for performing, here are some 'damage limitation' techniques: little strategies to use when things don't quite go according to plan when you are performing live.

Damage limitation

Note: You can use some of the following strategies when you are practising, too, since practising what to do when things go wrong will build your confidence in your own ability to handle any glitches in a live performance.

- Making mistakes is part of being human. The significance of a mistake often depends on how you react to it. If you pull a face or groan when you play a wrong note or, worst of all, stop playing, you will only make bigger what may have been a small glitch in an otherwise good performance. Drawing attention to errors in this way not only disturbs your concentration (perhaps causing you to make more mistakes) but can also affect your audience's confidence in you. So, keep going. Instead of allowing a stumble to put you off, let it make you even more determined to show what you are really capable of.

- Mistakes will always sound more severe and embarrassing to you, the performer, than they will to those listening (they are completely relaxed and therefore not as sensitive to these things as you). If you don't react to a slip in your playing and carry on as though nothing has happened, the chances are your audience won't even notice.

- If you make a mistake right at the start of a piece of music stop and, after taking a moment to compose yourself, begin again. This is the only time you should stop after making a mistake.

- If you make a mistake further on, don't draw attention to it; carry on playing as though nothing happened.

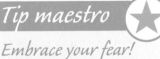

Tip maestro

Embrace your fear!

Expect *to feel nervous,* **accept** *that those butterflies and sweaty palms are going to come, but* **stay positive** *by reminding yourself that those feelings are helping you stay focused. That way you might even enjoy the rush of adrenaline!*

- If you are reading music and you lose your place (or have a memory lapse), just pick up from a point close to where you lost it and carry on. Don't waste time searching for where you should be and certainly don't stop to look.

Improvising

For techniques, advice and practice exercises in improvisation, see the supplementary material for this chapter at **www.jm-education.com**.

Glossary of musical concepts

National 5 concepts

STYLES

- ☐ **Aria** – a song, especially from an opera or oratorio.
- ☐ **Bothy ballad** – a traditional male Scottish folk song about hard work and working conditions (often involving farming).
- ☐ **Celtic rock** – rock music influenced by traditional Scottish and Irish music or with a distinctive Scottish or Irish feel. Sometimes this can be rock arrangements of traditional Scottish music, e.g. '**The Bonnie Banks of Loch Lomond**' by Runrig.
- ☐ **Chorus** – a large group of singers who perform together, often divided into parts for different voice ranges.
- ☐ **Classical** – the term used to describe music that is not part of folk or popular traditions, as well as music from the late eighteenth to early nineteenth centuries where careful attention to detail, formal structures (such as the sonata and symphony) and general high standards of musical excellence were the aim. Composers include Haydn, Mozart and Beethoven.
- ☐ **Gaelic Psalms** (or 'long tunes') – religious songs from the Western Isles of Scotland that can be sung slightly differently by individual members of a church congregation, creating an improvised feel, usually led by a solo male singer known as the precentor.
- ☐ **Gospel** – a style of religious singing that emerged in nineteenth-century America, influenced by the spirituals of black slaves and Protestant evangelical church music. In the twentieth century, gospel also became a popular song category not linked with religion.
- ☐ **Indian** – all styles of Indian music, including vocal music, Indian classical music and instrumental styles. Indian melodies are formed using special scales/modes called ragas and various set rhythmic patterns known as talas. It features the instruments of the sitar and tabla.
- ☐ **Minimalist** – a term first used in the early 1970s to describe music that uses simple, repetitive melodies and rhythms that are gradually extended by adding more and more of these simple 'layers' of music until a more complex structure develops.
- ☐ **Pibroch** – a term for more serious and complex solo highland bagpipe music – pibrochs use a theme and variation structure.
- ☐ **Symphony** – a large orchestral work, normally in three or four movements, which can last for up to an hour or more. A wide variety of musical structures, keys and emotions are often used in the musical journey of a symphony. Composers of symphonies include Mozart, Beethoven and Mahler.
- ☐ **Waulking song** – a traditional Scottish Gaelic song, usually with a repetitive rhythm, that was sung by people (mainly women) while they were doing tedious or repetitive work.

MELODY/HARMONY

☐ **Atonal** – a twentieth-century term describing music that is not tonal (e.g. is not in a key) and can freely use any notes; **Schoenberg**, **Webern** and **Berg** wrote some of the earliest atonal pieces.

☐ **Atonal music** – music that does not have a specific key but uses any note freely.

☐ **Chord progression** (**I, IV, V and VI in major keys**) – a sequence of chord changes. Chords I, IV, V and VI are built on the 1st, 4th, 5th and 6th notes of any scale; in major scales chords I, IV and V are always major, while chord VI is minor. In the key of C major, for example these chords would be C major (chord I), F major (chord IV), G major (chord V) and A minor (chord VI).

☐ **Chromatic scale** – a scale or a musical passage that moves in semitones (e.g. C C# D D# E F F# G G# A A# B C).

☐ **Cluster chord** – a bunch of adjacent notes played together (usually applies to piano music).

☐ **Contrary motion** – where two musical parts move in opposite directions.

☐ **Countermelody** – a second melody that complements the main melody and will usually also move in a different rhythm, as in counterpoint.

☐ **Descant** (voice) – a decorative extra part sung at a higher pitch above the main melody. Common in early sacred music and in choral music.

☐ **Glissando** – to slide smoothly between two notes that are some distance apart, with all the notes in between being played very rapidly.

☐ **Grace note** – an ornament where a rapid additional note or notes are used to decorate a melody.

☐ **Imperfect cadence** – two chords (such as I–V or II–V) that create the effect of a pause or 'comma' in a piece of music.

☐ **Inverted pedal** – a note that is sustained or constantly repeated in an upper part while other parts below it change.

☐ **Melismatic** – in vocal music, where several notes are sung to a single syllable, as in early religious plainsong.

☐ **Modulation** – when music changes from one key to another.

☐ **Perfect cadence** – two chords (V–I) that create the effect of an ending or 'full stop' to a phrase or entire piece of music. The Plagal cadence (IV–I) produces the same effect.

☐ **Pitch bend** – where a note is 'bent' away from its natural pitch by pulling down or pushing up a string on an instrument such as the guitar, sitar, violin or cello, or by moving the pitch bend control on a synthesiser or keyboard. Notes can be altered from a quarter tone to a full tone or sometimes more.

☐ **Semitone** – the musical interval (the distance between two notes) of half a tone, e.g. C to C#. This is the smallest distance between two notes in tonal music; every consecutive note on the piano keyboard is a semitone apart.

☐ **Syllabic** – in vocal music, where only one note is sung to every syllable; the opposite of melismatic music.

☐ **Tone** – a musical interval made up of two semitones, e.g. C to D.

☐ **Trill** – an ornament where two notes a semitone or a tone apart alternate rapidly with each other.

☐ **Whole-tone scale** – a scale that moves only in tones, e.g. C D E F# G# B♭ C.

RHYTHM/TEMPO

☐ **Compound time** (**6/8, 9/8, 12/8**) – a time signature where each beat is divisible by three. (See reference pages in the supplementary material at **www.jm-education.com**.)

☐ **Cross rhythms** – where the normal accents of a time signature are moved around to create different kinds of rhythms in a piece of music, or when separate parts play different rhythms at the same time.

☐ **Moderato** – an Italian term indicating that the music is to be played at a moderate speed.

☐ **Ritardando** – an Italian term indicating that the music should slow down gradually. Usually abbreviated to *rit.*

☐ **Rubato** – a term indicating that the tempo of a passage of music (or an entire piece) should be gently increased or decreased at will by the performer for an expressive effect.

TEXTURE/STRUCTURE/FORM

☐ **Alberti bass** – a broken chord pattern that is used as a bass accompaniment. The pattern is often: lowest note of chord – highest note of chord – middle note of chord – highest note of chord (e.g. C G E G).

☐ **Binary form** – a musical structure (A B), common in Baroque music, made up of two main sections, A and B, each of which is usually repeated. The B section is sometimes longer than the A section.

☐ **Coda** – a short 'ending' section that concludes a piece of music.

☐ **Contrapuntal** (**counterpoint**) – where two or more different musical parts (which sound complete in themselves) are played simultaneously to create a single, harmonious whole – a popular style in the Baroque period, but used by composers ever since.

☐ **Episode** – term given to a contrasting section in a rondo (see **rondo** below).

☐ **Ground bass** – a bass melody or motif that is constantly repeated with varying melodic lines above it.

☐ **Homophonic** – where voices or instruments sounding together move in the same rhythm.

☐ **Polyphonic** – where two or more voices or instruments sound together but have different rhythms. The term evolved in the sixteenth-century renaissance period.

☐ **Rondo** – a musical structure (A B A C A …) where the main theme (the A section) alternates with several new or contrasting sections of music (known as episodes).

☐ **Strophic** – a term used to describe vocal music in which different lyrics are sung to the same musical verse each time.

☐ **Walking bass** – a bass line where the note values and speed remain constant, as though walking steadily; a common technique in Baroque music but also used in jazz and boogie-woogie.

TIMBRE/DYNAMICS

☐ **A cappella** – a term originally meaning unaccompanied choral music, but now describes any vocal music unaccompanied by musical instruments. Examples include **Gregorian chant**, Choir music, Gospel, **Barbershop**, Rap and **Beat box**.

- **Arco** – 'bow': an instruction to players of bowed string instruments to go back to playing with the bow after a pizzicato section.
- **Baritone** – male voice between bass and tenor.
- **Bassoon** – a large woodwind instrument played by blowing into a double reed attached to a long, thin, curved metal tube. The **double bassoon** (sounding an octave lower than the standard instrument) is the lowest pitched member of the orchestral woodwind family. The bassoon is also used in some wind ensembles.
- **Bodhrán** – unpitched circular drum, held by one hand and rested on the player's leg while the other hand strikes the drum face (or wooden frame) with a wooden beater. Used as an accompaniment instrument, especially in Irish folk music.
- **Bongo drums** – small drums, normally played in pairs by striking with the hands. Commonly associated with Latin-American dance bands.
- **Castanets** – small unpitched wooden percussion instruments of Spanish origin, loosely bound together with a thin cord (which is looped around the thumbs) and held in the palms of the performer's hands. Castanets are played by the fingers of (usually female) flamenco dancers.
- **Clàrsach** – a small harp used in traditional Scottish and Irish folk music.
- **Con sordino** –'with the mute': an instruction to string and brass players to mute their sound.
- **Flutter-tonguing** – a technique used by wind players (especially on the flute) where the tongue rolls the letter 'r' to create a kind of **tremolo** effect.
- **French horn** – a brass instrument made from a tapering tube coiled into circles and widening out into a flared bell from which the sound escapes. It is played by blowing into a cup-shaped mouthpiece through the lips and using finger-operated valves. It has an ancient ancestry with many types, but the standard instrument has a central place as a medium to low-pitched instrument in the orchestral brass family.
- **Hi-hat cymbals** – unpitched percussion instruments consisting of two thin metal plates that are struck together by means of a foot pedal. Part of the standard drum kit used in pop, rock, jazz and blues bands.
- **Mezzo-soprano** – female voice between soprano and alto.
- **Oboe** – a hollow, cylindrical wind instrument made of hard wood that is played by blowing into a double reed attached to a thin metal tube. It is a principal member of the orchestral woodwind family.
- **Piccolo** – a miniature flute sounding an octave higher than the standard flute, often used in the orchestral woodwind family and some wind/military bands.
- **Pizzicato** – an instruction to string players to pluck the strings with the fingers instead of using the bow.
- **Reverb** – an electronic effect used to change the acoustic sound of amplified instruments (e.g. can make an instrument sound as though it is in a large concert hall even if it is being played in a small room).
- **Rolls** – term given to a trill performed on a drum.
- **Sitar** – a large and long-necked instrument of the lute family whose strings are plucked by the fingers and a wire plectrum attached to the index finger. Used in the classical music of India, Pakistan and Bangladesh, but it also features in some folk and popular music.

- **Tabla** – a pair of small drums (one treble and one bass) used widely in the classical music of India, Pakistan and Bangladesh.
- **Tuba** – the largest and lowest pitched member of the orchestral brass family. It is played by blowing into a cup-shaped mouthpiece through the lips and using finger-operated valves. The sound escapes through a large flared bell.
- **Viola** – four-stringed instrument usually played with a bow but sometimes plucked with a finger (pizzicato). Violas are a main orchestral instrument (the second highest pitched of the string family, slightly larger than the violin) but also feature in various ensemble groups (such as string quartets).

National 4 concepts

STYLES

- **African music** – several diverse musical styles feature in African music, with songs and chants unique to a vast number of regions or tribes. Many are based on short ideas that are improvised on. In one type a solo leader interacts with a larger group to create a vocal call and answer style. Instruments include a variety of drums, gongs, bells, rattles, xylophones, harps and harp-lutes, fiddles and an instrument known as a 'bow' because it is shaped like a hunting bow. There are also wind instruments similar to trumpets, horns, flutes and oboes, and a unique African instrument known as the 'sanza' or 'mbira', or 'thumb piano', made of a series of metal strips mounted on a resonant board that are plucked by the thumb. Complex rhythms and syncopation are common, using cross rhythms and **polyrhythms** – where several different rhythms are played simultaneously. In more recent times traditional African music has been combined with pop and disco styles to create musical **fusions**. African music is normally passed on to students who learn by ear rather than through music notation.
- **Baroque** – a term used to describe music from about 1600 to 1750 that is characterised by features such as contrast (e.g. contrasting dynamics, tempo etc.), walking bass and ornaments. The music often features the harpsichord. Famous Baroque composers include **J. S. Bach**, Handel and Vivaldi.
- **Concerto** – a large work, normally in three movements, for a solo instrument and orchestra – e.g. Vivaldi's '**The Four Seasons**' (for solo violin and orchestra), **Rodrigo's Concierto de Aranjuez** (for solo guitar and orchestra).
- **Mouth music** (**port-a-beul**) – an improvised vocal style used in place of musical instruments to accompany Scottish dances.
- **Opera** – a musical drama that is performed on stage with scenery (like a play) and singers who wear costumes and act out the roles of particular characters. The music (probably the most important part of any opera) is played by an orchestra placed in front of and below the stage (the pit). The two main kinds of opera are opera seria (serious opera) and opera buffa (comic opera). Famous opera composers include Mozart, Puccini and Verdi.
- **Ragtime** – a style of popular American music from the early 1900s, characterised by lively, often syncopated melodies, and a left-hand vamp in

strict rhythm. Most ragtime pieces were written for piano, and many of the more famous examples were composed by **Scott Joplin** (including '**The Entertainer**' and '**Maple Leaf Rag'**).

- [ ] **Rapping** – a popular style of African-American music where half-sung half-spoken melodies (often with improvised lyrics) are performed over a regular rhythmic accompaniment or beat.
- [ ] **Reggae** – originally appearing in Jamaica in the mid-1960s, reggae is now a popular style of urban dance music, characterised by accented upbeats or off-beats (syncopation).
- [ ] **Romantic** – the term used to describe the musical style of the nineteenth century where composers (such as Mahler, Wagner and **Berlioz**) created music that explored human feelings and experiences in greater depth than ever before. The music varied from dreamy, romantic or tranquil (such as piano miniatures by **Chopin** and **Debussy**) to the very loud and powerful (Wagner operas and orchestral works by Tchaikovsky). The orchestra increased in size and also used a wider variety of percussion.
- [ ] **Scots ballad** – a traditional Scottish folk song in which an unfortunate, sad or important historic story is told (e.g. a death, lost love, disaster or war).
- [ ] **Swing** – a style of lively popular jazz and big band dance music from the 1930s and 1940s. Pieces by **Glen Miller** are among the most famous from the time, as are songs sung by **Ella Fitzgerald**.

MELODY/HARMONY

- [ ] **Arpeggio** – a type of 'broken chord' where the notes of the chord are played one after the other (often in a rhythmic pattern) in an ascending or descending order instead of all together.
- [ ] **Broken chord** – when the notes of a chord are played separately rather than together.
- [ ] **Change of key** – when a piece of music changes (modulates) from one key to another.
- [ ] **Chord progression** (**chords I, IV and V in major keys**) – a sequence of chord changes. Chords I, IV and V are built on the 1st, 4th and 5th notes of any scale, and in major scales this always results in major chords. For example, in the key of C major, these chords would be C major (chord I), F major (chord IV) and G major (chord V).
- [ ] **Drone** – a constantly sustained note (normally a bass note), over which the main melody is played; bagpipes use at least one drone.
- [ ] **Major** and **minor** (**tonality**) – the key of a piece of music; a major key has a pleasant or 'happy' sound, and a minor key a serious or 'sad' sound.
- [ ] **Octave** – where the distance between two notes is 12 semitones, resulting in notes with the same name (e.g. A – A, C – C) but a different pitch. For example, if you play twelve consecutive keyboard keys (moving up or down) you will finish on a note with the same name (but different pitch) as the one you started on.
- [ ] **Ornament** – one or more 'decorative' notes added to a melody.
- [ ] **Pedal** – a note that is held (sustained) or constantly repeated while other parts above or below it change. Normally played in the bass part (bass pedal).

☐ **Pentatonic scale** – a scale that uses only five different notes (and no semitones) to make a particular sound (e.g. C E♭ F G B♭). Used in rock, jazz, blues and folk music.

☐ **Scale** – an ascending or descending succession of notes consisting of the different notes found in a particular key or mode (i.e. G A B C D E F# in the scale of G major).

☐ **Scat singing** – a style of jazz singing where meaningless words or syllables are improvised in a piece of music.

☐ **Vamp** – improvising a simple chord accompaniment (normally on the piano) in a piece of music. This accompaniment is often based on the repetitive pattern of a bass note followed by the chord.

RHYTHM/TEMPO

☐ **Accelerando** – gradually become faster.

☐ **Anacrusis** – the upbeat note (or notes) that comes before the first strong beat of a bar.

☐ **Andante** – a musical tempo meaning moderately slow or at a walking pace.

☐ **A tempo** – return to the original speed.

☐ **Compound time** – a time signature where the main beats are divisible by three, e.g. dotted quavers (6/8, 9/8, 12/8 time). (See Reference pages in the supplementary material at **www.jm-education.com**.)

☐ **Dotted rhythms** – rhythms with dots after the notes (dotted minims, dotted crotchets etc.), which add half the value of the original note (see National 5 Musical Literacy, page 21).

☐ **Jig** – a fast dance found in Scottish and Irish folk music, normally in compound time, e.g. 6/8, 9/8.

☐ **Rallentando** – gradually become slower.

☐ **Scotch snap** – a rhythm where a short note on the beat is followed by a longer one – ♪♩ – often used in Scottish music.

☐ **Simple time** – a time signature where the main beats are divisible by two, e.g. **crotchets** and **minims** (2/4, 3/4, 4/4 time). (See Reference pages in the supplementary material at **www.jm-education.com**.)

☐ **Strathspey** – a traditional Scottish dance in 4/4 time with a moderate tempo and characterised by a dotted rhythm, e.g. ♩♪ or a Scotch snap.

☐ **Syncopation** – where the accent is off the main beat and on a weaker beat (the up-beat, for example).

TEXTURE/STRUCTURE/FORM

☐ **Cadenza** – a complex section for the soloist (which shows his or her skill) near the end of a concerto movement or an aria. It is normally unaccompanied.

☐ **Canon** – a musical form where the first melody is imitated by another part (or parts) before the first melody is finished. This creates a texture where tunes overlap each other in a harmonious way.

☐ **Imitation** – when a musical phrase in one part is copied (imitated) in another part.

☐ **Middle 8** – an eight-bar instrumental section in a song that functions as a link between the verse and chorus.

☐ **Ternary form** – a musical structure made up of three main sections, A B A, where the B section normally provides some musical contrast and the second A section can either be an exact or altered repeat of the first A section. Sometimes the structure is A A B A.

☐ **Theme and variation** – a musical form where a theme is played and then followed by a set of variations based on that theme. The variations normally include changes to the speed, key, rhythm etc. of the main theme.

☐ **Verse and chorus** – a structure used in songs where verses whose lyrics change with each new verse alternate with a (normally) livelier chorus whose lyrics stay the same each time.

TIMBRE/DYNAMICS

☐ **Alto** – female voice below soprano or sometimes a high male voice.

☐ **Backing vocals** – the singers who accompany the lead vocalist.

☐ **Bass** – the lowest pitched male voice.

☐ **Bass drum** – a large drum made from a wooden cylindrical shell over which the playing surface or membrane (made from plastic or animal hide) is stretched. When used in the orchestra (where it is the largest unpitched percussion instrument in the percussion family) it is struck with a hand-held felt-headed beater, but when used as part of a drum kit in modern rock and pop groups this beater is operated by a foot pedal.

☐ **Bass guitar** – a large guitar with four heavy, low pitched strings that create a deep, resonant sound; these can be plucked with the fingers or a plectrum.

☐ **Brass band** – a band in which different kinds of brass instruments such as cornet, horn and euphonium are played. May also include percussion.

☐ **Cello** – large four-stringed instrument played with a bow or plucked with a finger (pizzicato). This is a main orchestral instrument (the second largest and second lowest pitched of the string family) but is also used in ensemble groups such as string quartets and played solo.

☐ **Clarinet** – a hollow, cylindrical wind instrument played by blowing into a mouthpiece that has a single reed. It has several types, the most common being the **B flat clarinet**, which is a member of the orchestral woodwind family, but the clarinet is also used in ensembles, dance bands and jazz music.

☐ **Cymbals** – unpitched percussion instrument comprising two round plates of thin metal that are struck together. In the orchestra, large hand-held cymbals are common, but sometimes a single suspended cymbal, struck with a beater (drumstick), is used. In rock, pop and (especially) jazz bands, smaller types of suspended cymbals are used as part of the drum kit; these are either operated by a foot pedal or struck with drumsticks.

☐ **Distortion** – an electronic effect used on amplified instruments (particularly electric guitar) that creates a 'dirty', distorted sound that is often used in rock and heavy metal music.

☐ **Double bass** – large four-stringed instrument played with a bow or the fingers. Although a main orchestral instrument (the largest and lowest pitched of the string family), the double bass is also popular in jazz ensembles.

☐ **Flute** – a hollow, cylindrical wind instrument made of wood or (more commonly) metal whose sound is produced by a column of air blown into the mouth hole. A high pitched (soprano) member of the orchestral woodwind family, the flute also features in military/wind bands, ensembles, and jazz and Latin-American music.

☐ **Glockenspiel** – a pitched percussion instrument consisting of a standing frame on which a number of tuned metal bars of different length are arranged like a piano keyboard and struck with beaters.

☐ **Güiro** – a small unpitched percussion instrument made from a long notched board that is rubbed to create a rasping sound. It is used sometimes in the orchestra and in Latin-American, folk and popular bands.

☐ **Harp** – a musical instrument with a large frame and strings that are perpendicular to the soundboard or resonator. There are several types of harp, including the smaller **clàrsach**, but the modern concert harp has 47 strings, which produce a mellow, resonant sound by being strummed, plucked or struck with the fingers. It also has pedals, which allow the pitch of each string to be raised by two semitones.

☐ **Harpsichord** – a keyboard instrument whose sound is produced by strings that are plucked each time a key is struck. The harpsichord was very popular both as a solo and accompaniment instrument in the Baroque period.

☐ **Muted** – dampening the sound produced by an instrument to make it quieter or to alter the sound; this can be done with the hand on some instruments (such as guitar and French horn), or by using a special device known as a mute (on orchestral stringed instruments and brass instruments).

☐ **Panpipes** – a hand-held instrument made from small pipes of varying length that are joined together, played by blowing over the top end of the pipes while the bottom ends are stopped. Panpipes are an ancient instrument but still used in the folk music of South America (especially the Andes), Romania, Oceania and Burma.

☐ **Recorder** – a woodwind instrument that dates back to the fourteenth century. There have been several types, tuned to different pitches, but the most common are the descant, treble, tenor and bass recorders.

☐ **Saxophone** – a hollow wind instrument made of metal (normally brass) with a cone-shaped interior, which is played by blowing into a mouthpiece that has a single reed. Type and size vary, but the most commonly played saxophone is the larger instrument with a U-bend, supported on the performer with a strap. It is used in wind/military and dance bands, jazz and pop music, and in some orchestral music from the Romantic period onwards.

☐ **Snare drum** – a drum with a series of metal springs stretched below its striking surface (membrane) to produce a particular sound when struck by drumsticks. It is an unpitched percussion instrument often used as part of a 'drum kit' in modern groups, as well as in jazz and wind/military bands and occasionally in the orchestra as a 'side drum'.

☐ **Soprano** – the highest pitched female voice.

☐ **Tambourine** – a hand-held unpitched percussion instrument made from a wooden frame into which metal jingles are inserted, and covered on one side by a stretched piece of plastic or skin that is normally struck with the hand or thumb.

☐ **Tenor** – a male voice pitched higher than bass and lower than alto.

☐ **Timpani** – several large drums played by striking with two beaters or drumsticks, the timpani are pitched percussion instruments and one of the most important members of the orchestral percussion family.

- ☐ **Triangle** – small unpitched percussion instrument made from a steel rod formed into a triangular shape (open at one corner) and struck with a small metal beater. It has a bright, resonant sound and is normally used in wind/military bands and the orchestra.
- ☐ **Trombone** – a large brass instrument made from a long hollow tube gradually widening out into a cone (the bell) from which the sound escapes. The trombone is played by blowing into its cup-shaped mouthpiece through the lips and using a hand operated telescopic slide that varies the length of the tube and changes the notes. It is used in brass, wind/military and dance bands and jazz music, and is the third-highest pitched (tenor) member of the orchestral brass family.
- ☐ **Trumpet** – a brass instrument made from a hollow tube widening out to a cone (the bell) from which the sound escapes. The trumpet is played by blowing into its cup-shaped mouthpiece through the lips and using three finger-operated valves. It has been around since ancient times and today there are several different types (of varying pitches) used in brass, wind/military and dance bands and jazz music, and it has a central place as a high-pitched member of the orchestral brass family.
- ☐ **Violin** – four-stringed instrument played with a bow but sometimes plucked with a finger (pizzicato). Violins are a main orchestral instrument (the smallest and highest pitched of the string family), where they are often divided into two sections, but they also feature in various ensemble groups (such as string quartets) and are played solo.
- ☐ **Wind/military band** – a band of woodwind, brass and percussion musicians who often play brisk military music including marches (such as those by **John Philip Sousa**).
- ☐ **Xylophone** – a pitched percussion instrument consisting of a large standing frame on which a number of flat wooden bars of different length are laid out rather like a piano keyboard; these bars have cords going through them that are attached to tube resonators that produce the sound.

National 3 concepts

STYLES

- ☐ **Blues** – an improvised African-American folk music whose name refers to the often melancholy nature of the music and the 'blue' (discordant) notes used. Blues is based on chord progressions that last for 8, 12 or 32 bars (the most common being 12 bar blues) over which a melody normally based on the blues scale is played or sung.
- ☐ **Jazz** – an improvised style of music developed by African-Americans in the early twentieth century that often uses lively swing rhythms and bent pitches (discordant notes used to 'colour' the music).
- ☐ **Latin-American** – a style that blends different kinds of music from several cultures, including Spain, the Caribbean and South America. One of its most popular versions is lively South-American jazz.

☐ **Musical** – a popular twentieth-century form of musical theatre, developed from comic opera, with light-hearted, romantic or humorous plots and catchy, up-beat songs as well as spectacular dances and spoken text. Composers of musicals include **George Gershwin**, **Stephen Sondheim** and **Andrew Lloyd Webber**.

☐ **Pop** – a style of music that uses modern sounds and song lyrics (words) that are normally popular with the mass public, particularly the younger generation.

☐ **Rock** – a popular modern style of music that developed from rock 'n' roll. Rock music often uses 'heavier' lyrics and more driving beats than pop music even though both styles use electric instruments, drums and amplified singing.

☐ **Rock 'n' roll** – a style of dance music from mid-1950s America that developed from rhythm-and-blues. **Elvis Presley** was one of the most famous rock 'n' roll singers of all time.

☐ **Scottish** – music linked closely with Scotland and traditional (early) Scottish styles such as the reel, jig, Strathspey, mouth music, bothy ballad etc.

MELODY/HARMONY

☐ **Ascending** – where the music becomes higher in pitch as it progresses.

☐ **Chord** – three or more notes played at the same time. All common chords such as C, G, D, Am, Em are made up of the 1st, 3rd and 5th notes of their scale. For example, the chord of C major has the notes, C, E and G (the 1st, 3rd and 5th notes of the scale). See Scales and key signatures, page 20.

☐ **Chord change** – when a chord, and therefore the harmony, changes in a piece.

☐ **Descending** – where the music becomes lower in pitch as it progresses.

☐ **Discord** (or **dissonance**) – notes or chords that sound harsh or clashing.

☐ **Improvisation** – when music is made up on the spot, often using the notes in a particular scale (major, pentatonic etc.) in no particular order to invent a melody.

☐ **Leap** (**leaping**) – where the music moves in big jumps.

☐ **Question and answer** – two musical phrases where the first (the question) sounds as though it is being 'answered' (the answer) by the second – as in speech.

☐ **Repetition** – where a passage or a whole section of music is repeated.

☐ **Sequence** – when a passage of music is repeated at a higher or lower pitch.

☐ **Step** (**stepwise**) – where the music moves in small steps rather than big jumps.

RHYTHM/TEMPO

☐ **Accent** – a musical symbol > written above or below notes or chords that are to be played slightly louder.

☐ **Accented** – a musical note, phrase, chord or passage that contains accents.

☐ **Adagio** – a musical term meaning 'slow'.

☐ **Allegro** – a musical term meaning 'lively', or 'quite fast'.

☐ **Bar** – the 'compartments' on the musical stave that separate notes into a set number of beats; e.g. 2, 3 and 4 beats per bar.

- ☐ **Beat/pulse** – the steady main pulse in a piece of music.
- ☐ **Drum fill** – a passage of drum beats used before the start or at the end of a musical phrase to 'fill' the gaps.
- ☐ **Faster** – when a piece of music speeds up, often indicated by the musical term *accel.* (*accelerando*).
- ☐ **March** – a musical composition in duple metre (two main beats per bar) that is intended to be marched to.
- ☐ **Off the beat** – where the stress or accent is off the beat (on the 'up-beat', for example – as in syncopation). When there are four beats in a bar, beats 2 and 4 are off the beat.
- ☐ **On the beat** – where the stress or accent is on the main beat(s).
- ☐ **Pause** – where the music stops briefly; sometimes indicated by a **fermata** – a musical symbol ⌒ written over a note, chord or rest to indicate that the player(s) should pause at that point.
- ☐ **Reel** – a lively Scottish dance in duple metre (two beats per bar) that moves in fast, smooth quavers. Also common in Ireland and North America.
- ☐ **Repetition** – where a passage or section of music is repeated.
- ☐ **Slower** – when a piece of music slows down, often indicated by the musical term *rall.* (*rallentando*).
- ☐ **Waltz** – a moderate tempo dance in triple metre (three main beats per bar).

TEXTURE/STRUCTURE/FORM

- ☐ **Accompanied** – where the most important melody or solo in a piece of music has another instrument or instruments playing along with it (e.g. a song with piano accompaniment).
- ☐ **Harmony** – where notes are combined/played at the same time to produce satisfactory sounds and create texture in a piece of music (e.g. chord accompaniment, countermelody).
- ☐ **Octave** – when all the parts in a piece of music are played or sung together but one octave apart (in octaves) – e.g. a violin plays the notes C, D and B, and a cello plays the same notes (C, D and B) but one octave lower in pitch.
- ☐ **Ostinato** – the constant repetition of the same musical phrase, rhythm pattern or chords.
- ☐ **Repetition** – where a passage or section of music is repeated, perhaps as an ostinato or riff.
- ☐ **Riff** – a short musical phrase of around two to four bars long that is repeated regularly throughout a piece of music (especially in jazz, rock and pop music).
- ☐ **Round** – a musical form where a short main theme is repeated in other parts at staggered intervals to create an overlapping texture (as in the children's song, 'Row, Row, Row Your Boat').
- ☐ **Solo** – a section of music or a whole piece performed by just one musician.
- ☐ **Unaccompanied** – where no other instruments play along with the main melody or instrument in a piece of music; the opposite of accompanied.
- ☐ **Unison** – when certain parts in a piece of music are played or sung together at exactly the same pitch and with the same rhythm – e.g. singing in unison rather than in harmony.

TIMBRE/DYNAMICS

☐ **Accordion** – a portable reed organ (attached to the body with two straps) that has treble piano keys (or buttons) played by the right hand and bass buttons played by the left. Air is pumped into what has become this traditional Scottish instrument by bellows operated by the player. Popular in Scottish dance bands, Scottish folk groups and ceilidh bands.

☐ **Acoustic guitar** – large bodied plucked string instrument with frets and steel strings. Can also be strummed.

☐ **Bagpipes** – wind instrument used in traditional Scottish music consisting of a tube and mouthpiece attached to an air bag (which is pumped by the player's arm) and a set of pipes from which the sound is produced. Individual notes are selected by the fingers on a hand-held device called a chanter.

☐ **Blowing** – the method of producing sound on any wind instrument (e.g. flute, trumpet, recorder) by using the breath.

☐ **Bowing** – the method of producing sound on a string instrument (violin, cello, double bass etc.) by drawing a bow over the strings.

☐ **Choir** (choral) – music where voice is the main instrument. Choral music involves a choir (a large group of singers), which can be made up of male voices only, female voices only, male and female voices, or children's voices (youth choir).

☐ **Drum kit** – a selection of different drums and cymbals set together and played by beaters or 'drum sticks' by a performer who sits in the centre of the kit.

☐ **Electric guitar** – amplified plucked string instrument with a solid body and steel strings. Can also be strummed.

☐ **Fiddle** – the word used for a violin when it is used to play certain kinds of music, especially folk music and traditional Scottish and Irish music.

☐ **Folk group** – a band of musicians who play folk music. In Scottish folk music such a group would play instruments such as fiddle, penny whistle, accordion and guitar.

☐ **Legato** – smooth notes or chords with no silences in between (the opposite of staccato).

☐ **Orchestra** – a large group of musicians who play a selection of instruments grouped into four main 'families': woodwind, brass, percussion (tuned and untuned) and strings. Music can be either written especially for orchestra (e.g. a symphony) or arranged for it, but in all cases the orchestra is led by a conductor who dictates the speed, dynamics and overall interpretation of a piece, and generally makes sure everyone plays well together.

☐ **Organ** – although technically a wind instrument because air produces the sound through large pipes (unless it is a much smaller electric organ), an organ is a keyboard instrument with black and white keys set out in semitones and played by the musician's fingers; it also has foot pedals and stops (buttons that alter the volume and the type of sound produced).

☐ **Piano** – keyboard instrument with black and white keys set out in semitones that are played by a seated musician's fingers.

☐ **Plucking** – a method of producing sound on any string instrument by striking the strings with the fingers or (on guitars and banjo) a plectrum (a small triangular shaped object).

☐ **Scottish dance band** – a group, consisting of instruments such as piano, accordion, fiddle and drums, who play traditional Scottish music.

☐ **Staccato** – short, detached notes or chords.

☐ **Steel band** – a group of musicians who play steel drums – tuned percussion instruments that are made from oil drums. These bands began in the 1930s in the West Indies.

☐ **Striking** (**hitting**) – when an instrument is hit (with the hand or a beater – such as a drum stick) to produce a sound.

☐ **Strumming** – a method of producing sound on string instruments such as the guitar and banjo by quickly drawing the fingers or a plectrum (a small triangular shaped object) across the strings.

☐ **Voice** (vocal) – the creation of musical notes using the voice, as in songs.

Answers to specimen listening test

Question 1

CD track 1

a) ☑ Musical

b) *Accompanied voice* or *verse and chorus*

CD track 2

c) ☑ Concerto

d) *Trill*

CD track 3

e) ☑ Symphony

f) *Staccato. Arco* also acceptable

Question 2

CD track 4

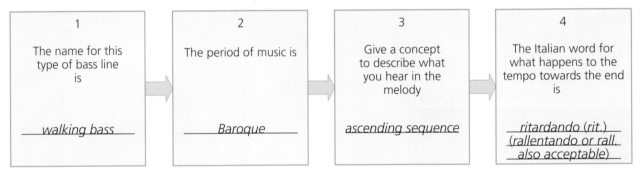

1	2	3	4
The name for this type of bass line is	The period of music is	Give a concept to describe what you hear in the melody	The Italian word for what happens to the tempo towards the end is
walking bass	*Baroque*	*ascending sequence*	*ritardando (rit.) (rallentando or rall. also acceptable)*

Question 3

CD track 5

Moderato (or Andante)

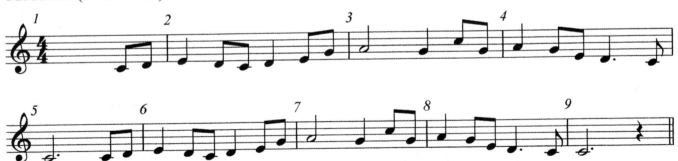

a) Name the key of this excerpt. *C major*

b) Insert the time signature in the correct place (see musical notation above).

c) Name the lowest and highest notes in the excerpt. *C and C*

d) Write an Italian term at the correct place to indicate the tempo (see diagram above).

e) How many different note values (e.g. crotchet, quaver) does the note **D** have in the excerpt? *Three (quaver, crotchet and dotted crotchet)*

f) Complete bar 6 by inserting the missing notes (see musical notation above).

Question 4

CD track 6

a) ☑ Aria

CD track 7

b) *Reggae*

CD track 8

c) ☑ Soprano

CD track 9

d) ☑

I	VI	IV	V
G	Em	C	D

CD track 10

e) ☑ Syllabic
☑ Homophonic

CD track 11

f) ☑ Syncopation
g) *Timpani*

Question 5

CD track 12

		Tick
Solo instrument	Flute	
	Bagpipes	
	Accordion	✓
Accompanying instrument	Snare drum	✓
	Clàrsach	
	Bodhrán	
Scottish dance	Waltz	
	Reel	
	Strathspey	✓
Tempo	Andante	
	Adagio	
	Allegro	✓

Question 6

CD track 13

There are **three** beats in each bar.

A small group of instruments from the *string* family join in the melody.

The excerpt is in *ternary* form.

Question 7

CD track 14

a) ☑ Latin-American

Reason (possible answers): *Latin percussion; Latin rhythms; bongo drums; Spanish vocals*

CD track 15

b) ☑ Romantic

Reason (possible answers): *large orchestra; expressive; dramatic; sudden dynamic contrasts; use of chromaticism; prominent percussion (side/snare drum, cymbals)*

Question 8

CD track 16

ROUGH WORK (example)

Rhythm/tempo	*Andante. Adagio. 3 beats in the bar (or 3/4 or triple metre)*
Melody/harmony	*Minor key. Staccato strings enter eventually, playing an ostinato, followed by woodwind with strings playing descending figures.* *Bass pedal*
Instruments/voices	*Male voices, unaccompanied. Chorus. Homophonic. A cappella. Orchestral accompaniment follows. Ostinato accompaniment. Legato voices with staccato strings. Timpani rolls.*
Dynamics	*pp at start. Crescendo builds to ff*

FINAL ANSWER (example)

Andante. 3 beats in a bar (or 3/4 or triple metre). Minor key. Ostinato strings and woodwind. Timpani. Chorus of unaccompanied male voices (a cappella). Homophonic. pp at the start, with a slowly building crescendo; legato voices are eventually accompanied by staccato strings; a short ritardando follows as the crescendo builds to ff. Orchestra enters. Strings play descending musical figures, accompanied by woodwind and a bass pedal. Timpani rolls.

CD track list

CD track	Title	Composer (Performers)	Recording co.	Page
1	**Tomorrow** (from the musical 'Annie')	Music: Charles Strouse; lyrics: Martin Charnin (Emma Isola)	**Sotogrande International School**	22
2	**Piano Concerto no. 21 in C Major, K467, 'Elvira Madigan.'** (movement 2, *Andante*)	**Mozart** (Peter Lang, Capella Istropolitana Orchestra, Conductor: Stephen Gunzenhauser)	**Naxos**	23
3	**Symphony no. 9** (movement 2, *Molto vivace*)	**Beethoven** (London Philharmonic Orchestra, conductor: Klaus Tennstedt)	**Warner Chappell**	23
4	**Air on a G string**	**J. S. Bach** (Scottish Chamber Orchestra directed by Jaime Laredo)	The Orchid Series. Innovative Music Productions Ltd. A division of **The Pickwick Group Ltd**	23
5	**The Salley Gardens**	**Traditional**	**jm-education**	24
6	**La Donna e Mobile**, (from 'Rigoletto')	**Verdi** (Nürnberg Symphony Orchestra – Hans Zanotelli, Conductor, Rudolf Knoll, Baritone)	**Countdown Media**	25
7	**Go Tell it on the Mountain**	**Traditional** (Bob Marley and the Wailers)	**Blue Mountain Music**	25
8	**Music for a While**	**Purcell – Dryden** (vocalist: Elizabeth Ritchie; piano: Jennifer Purvis)	The Orchid Series Innovative Music Productions Ltd. A division of **The Pickwick Group Ltd**	25
9	**Listening Test Example** (Question 4d)	**Joe McGowan**	**jm-education**	25
10	**Sailors' Chorus** (from 'The Flying Dutchman')	**Richard Wagner** (Radio Symphony Orchestra and Choir Ljubljana, conducted by Marko Munih)	'Richard Wagner' (Masters of the Millennium series) **Point Classics UK Ltd, London**. Permission granted from **ONE MEDIA iP Ltd**	25

CD track	Title	Composer (Performers)	Recording co.	Page
11	**Sailors' Chorus** (from 'The Flying Dutchman')	**Richard Wagner** (Radio Symphony Orchestra and Choir Ljubljana, conducted by Marko Munih)	'Richard Wagner' (Masters of the Millennium series) **Point Classics UK Ltd, London**. Permission granted from **ONE MEDIA iP Ltd**	26
12	**Strathspey Écosse**	**Traditional**		26
13	**Menuet** (from 'Water Music' – suite in F major)	**G. F. Handel** (City of London Sinfonia, directed by Richard Hickox)	The Orchid Series. Innovative Music Productions Ltd. A division of T**he Pickwick Group Ltd**	27
14	**Cancion para un niño**	**Ray Barretto** (Ricky Gonzalez, Carlitos Soto)	**Fania Records**. Permission granted from **Mr Bongo Worldwide Ltd**	27
15	**Emperor's Waltz, op. 437**	**Richard Strauss** (Vienna Opera Orchestra, conducted by Peter Falk)	**Countdown Media**	27
16	**Pilgrim's Chorus** 'Beglückt darf nun'	**Richard Wagner** (Radio Symphony Orchestra and Choir Ljubljana, conducted by Marko Munih)	'Richard Wagner' Masters of the Millennium series. **Point Classics UK Ltd, London**. Permission granted from **ONE MEDIA iP Ltd**	27
17	Instrumental composing example	**Joe McGowan**	**jm-education**	36
18	Instrumental composing example	**Joe McGowan**	**jm-education**	38
19	Instrumental composing example	**Joe McGowan**	**jm-education**	41
20	Instrumental composing example	**Joe McGowan**	**jm-education**	42
21	Instrumental composing example	**Joe McGowan**	**jm-education**	43
22	Instrumental composing example	**Joe McGowan**	**jm-education**	45
23	Vocal composing example	**Joe McGowan**	**jm-education**	50

CD track	Title	Composer (Performers)	Recording co.	Page
24	Vocal composing example	**Joe McGowan**	**jm-education**	50
25	Vocal composing example	**Joe McGowan**	**jm-education**	51
26	Vocal composing example	**Joe McGowan**	**jm-education**	53
27	Vocal composing example	**Joe McGowan**	**jm-education**	53
28	Vocal composing example	**Joe McGowan**	**jm-education**	53
29	'I'm Arising'. Example from supplementary songwriting workshop at **www.jm-education.com**	**Chloe Lawrence**	**jm-education**	—
30	'Latin Dance'. Example from supplementary composing workshop at **www.jm-education.com**	**Joe McGowan**	**jm-education**	—

Blank manuscript paper

Blank listening observation chart

Style	Composer/ performer	Compositions/ performances	Concepts/instruments/ other characteristics

Have you seen our full range of revision and exam practice resources?

ESSENTIAL SQA EXAM PRACTICE

National 5 | **Higher**

Practice questions and papers

- ✓ Dozens of questions covering every question type and topic
- ✓ Two practice papers that mirror the real SQA exams
- ✓ Advice for answering different question types and achieving better grades

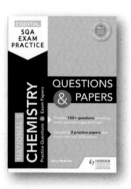 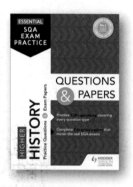

NEED to KNOW

Higher

Quick-and-easy revision

- ✓ Bullet-pointed summaries of the essential content
- ✓ Quick exam tips on common mistakes and things to remember
- ✓ Short 'Do you know?' knowledge-check questions

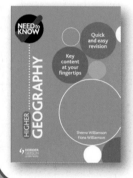 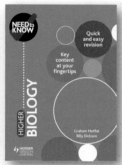 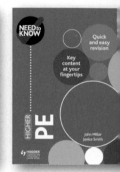

✓ How to Pass

National 5 | **Higher**

Scotland's most popular revision guides

- ✓ Comprehensive notes covering all the course content
- ✓ In-depth guidance on how to succeed in the exams and assignments
- ✓ Exam-style questions to test understanding of each topic

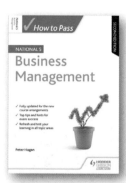 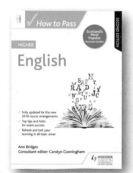 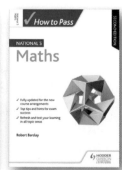

Our revision and exam practice resources are available across a whole range of subjects including the sciences, English, maths, business and social subjects.

Find out more and order online at **www.hoddergibson.co.uk**

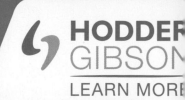

HODDER GIBSON
LEARN MORE